NURSING RESEARCH IN ACTION

◆ NURSING RESEARCH IN ACTION

Developing Basic Skills

Philip Burnard and Paul Morrison

*Lecturers in Nursing Studies,
University of Wales College of Medicine,
Cardiff*

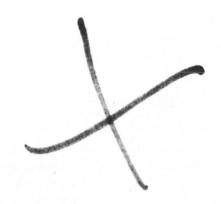

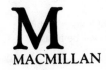

MACMILLAN

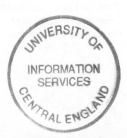

First published in 1990 by
THE MACMILLAN PRESS LTD
Houndmills, Basingstoke, Hampshire RG21 2XS
and London
Companies and representatives
throughout the world

ISBN 0–333–49563–2

A catalogue record for this book is available
from the British Library.

Printed in Hong Kong

Reprinted 1991, 1992

Acknowledgements

The authors would like to thank Bunny le Roux, Principal Lecturer,
Department of Applied Statistics and Operational Research, Sheffield
City Polytechnic for permission to reproduce the statistical exercise in
Chapter 8; and the Science and Engineering Research Council for
permission to adapt material from *An Approach to Good Supervisory
Practice* (1983).

   Every effort has been made to trace all the copyright holders, but if
any have been inadvertently overlooked the publishers will be pleased
to make the necessary arrangement at the first opportunity.

for Sally, Aaron and Rebecca
and
Franziska, Sarah and Maeve

◆CONTENTS

✦FOREWORD

Philip Burnard and Paul Morrison invite the novice to develop basic
research skills by undertaking a series of exercises which explore the
stages of conceptualising, planning, carrying out and writing a
research project. This book is aimed at absolute beginners and will be
a necessary companion for Project 2000 students or for nurses
undertaking research as part of the requirements for post-registration
certificates. Teachers who may have to introduce students to research
and who have limited experience will also find the book useful.
Although addressed to those unfamiliar with the research process it
should also be of use to more advanced students who might be
tempted to jump into a project without going through the essential
clarification and planning stages or who might want to try out some
unfamiliar method.

The authors' approach is grounded in their experience of teaching
and supervising students preparing research dissertations at the
undergraduate and masters level. Much of the material is drawn from
recent nursing research literature.

However, suggested reading is not just nursing based but draws
from a wider field and should encourage even those for whom a
research project is a 'one-off' to consider theory and methods of other
disciplines.

Methods which are often inadequately explained in research papers
or described in complex terms in research monographs are presented
in the form of a DIY manual, with exercises and information boxes,
which enables the student to perform the necessary operations as well
as to try out each of the skills under supervision and through that
experience to gain an understanding of the ideas and concepts
involved.

The handbook can be used as the basis for individual or group
work. Student/supervisor contracts, sources of information, reviewing
the literature, referencing, going to the ethical committee, the use of
diagrams and basic descriptive statistics are all dealt with through the

medium of practical exercises which move the student from one stage of the research process to the next. The pace is fast with emphasis on clearing a series of small but significant hurdles with the finishing line of the final report or published paper always kept in sight.

The authors offer no short cuts to the development of research expertise. But they do much to de-mystify the process and make the steps accessible to any student who is prepared to make the effort to go along with them.

Jillian MacGuire
RCN Professor of Nursing Research
University of Wales College of Medicine

◆ ABOUT THE AUTHORS

Philip Burnard

Philip is a lecturer in nursing at the University of Wales College of Medicine and an honorary lecturer at the Institute for Higher Professional Education of Health Care Professions, Utrecht, Netherlands. His research projects have explored experiential learning in nursing and nurses' perceptions of their interpersonal skills. He has contributed numerous articles to the nursing journals and is author of *Learning Human Skills: a Guide for Nurses, Professional and Ethical Issues in Nursing: the Code of Professional Conduct* (with C. M. Chapman), *Counselling Skills for Health Professionals* and *Teaching Interpersonal Skills: a Handbook of Experiential Learning for Health Professionals*. He is particularly interested in the fields of counselling, spirituality and nurse education. Philip is married with two children and lives in Caerphilly, South Wales.

Paul Morrison

Paul is also a lecturer in nursing at the University of Wales College of Medicine. He has undertaken various research projects, including those that look at consumer satisfaction in psychiatric care, seclusion in the management of disturbed behaviour and nurses' perceptions of their interpersonal skills. His current research work is concerned with how nurses and patients construe the nature of caring. He has contributed articles to the nursing press and he has a particular interest in the application of psychology to practice. Paul is married with two children and lives in Barry, South Wales.

◆ INTRODUCTION

Research is a means of understanding, assessing and evaluating what we do as nurses. It can help us to plan for the future. It can be exciting and satisfying. It can also be hard work. If you are just beginning to study research, this book will help you think about the stages of the research process. It will also help you develop basic research skills. Whilst research is never a clear–cut and tidy process, one alternative to either giving up or being overwhelmed by the task is to develop *structure*. In this book we develop a structured approach to research.

The book aims to make nursing research possible for those who are just setting out. The book offers a series of exercises and as you follow them you will begin to learn how to do research yourself. We suggest that after you have finished working through this book you do a piece of research yourself. However, we do not suggest that you do it alone. Research is often hard work and uses a whole range of skills. It is not something to be rushed into.

It is not our intention that this book should stand alone. It can be used as a guide alongside other texts on research and should be used with a tutor and with other nursing colleagues.

We are both nurses and both teach nursing and research methods. Driven by the idea that there is no better way to learn to do something than by doing it, we have undertaken a number of research projects. We have also supervised students and have learned, for instance, that there is no one 'right' way to do research. We have also learned that one of the best ways to learn research is to do it. We hope that this book will allow you to sample various aspects of the research process as a means of building up a range of research skills.

The book may be used on its own as a learning package. A nurse working through the book can do the exercises and follow up the approaches through reference to the books and articles recommended throughout the text. The extended recommended reading list at the back of the book and the compendium of research resources will be further aids.

The book may also be used as part of a student-centred learning programme. Nurse educators realise that people learn at different speeds and that their learning needs vary. So the book can be tailored to suit the varying needs of the people using it. For some, it will help to work right through the book as an introduction to research methods. For others, it will be more appropriate to select certain chapters relating to specific skills.

The book unfolds logically to cover all the stages of the research process. As it does this, a wide and varied range of references is offered so the book can be a rich source of reference for anyone who wants to become familiar with a broad view of the research literature. Examples of research projects are drawn not only from nursing but from the whole range of social sciences. We feel that it is important that nurses sample and explore all sorts of approaches to doing research.

Many of the information boxes can serve as the means by which ideas are sparked off or the next stage of a research project is planned. The references offered throughout the book and in the bibliography will also be useful in gaining new leads and developing thoughts and plans.

The book is not just theoretical in nature. It invites the reader to complete a range of exercises to reinforce learning. It may be used in a group setting with discussion following each exercise. If the book is used in this way, it is recommended that the tutor or facilitator should appreciate that each student will tend to find different results at the end of each exercise. Plenty of time should be allowed for the completion of the exercises and about an hour should be provided for discussion. It is suggested that the experiential learning cycle on p. 3 is studied in order to make full use of the exercises.

An experiential learning cycle applied to the exercises in this book.

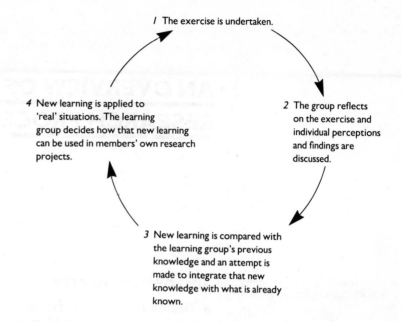

I The exercise is undertaken.

2 The group reflects on the exercise and individual perceptions and findings are discussed.

3 New learning is compared with the learning group's previous knowledge and an attempt is made to integrate that new knowledge with what is already known.

4 New learning is applied to 'real' situations. The learning group decides how that new learning can be used in members' own research projects.

The book offers an exploratory approach to most aspects of the research cycle. Quantitative and qualitative methods of doing research are addressed as is a variety of ways of collecting and analysing data. The reader is encouraged to draw up a research proposal, identify the data collection methods and methods of analysis. He/she is then directed towards writing the project. A series of 'information boxes' is offered throughout the text to illuminate certain aspects of the topics under discussion. At the end of the book there is a compendium containing further information. Overall, the book should serve as a practical introduction to research in nursing.

Philip Burnard
Paul Morrison
Cardiff
March 1990

1 ◆ AN OVERVIEW OF THE RESEARCH PROCESS

WHAT YOU NEED TO READ

Bell, J. (1987). *Doing Your Research Project: A Guide For First-Time Researchers in Education and Social Science*, Open University, Milton Keynes.

Cormack, D. F. S. (ed) (1984). *The Research Process in Nursing*, Blackwell, Oxford; chapters 1 and 2.

Skevington, S. (ed) (1984). *Understanding Nurses: The Social Psychology of Nursing*, Wiley, Chichester; chapter 1.

Treece, E. W. and Treece, J. W. (1982). *Elements of Research in Nursing*, 3rd Edition, C. V. Mosby, St Louis; chapter 2.

AIMS OF THIS CHAPTER

- To identify definitions of research;
- To identify examples of different sorts of research;
- To outline the stages of the research process;
- To help you plan your research project in a structured and methodical way.

INTRODUCTION

Research has been defined in various ways and in this chapter you will be exploring some of those definitions. Almost all research goes through certain stages. If you can develop the skill of breaking down your project into manageable chunks you will find it easier to control and to perform. The first part of the chapter invites you to think about research and the second part offers you a way of identifying the stages that make up the research process.

1 DEFINITIONS OF RESEARCH

By the end of this section you will have discovered:

- how to define research;
- the meanings or usage of certain words.

INFORMATION BOX

Some definitions of research

'Careful search or inquiry *after* or *for* or *into*; endeavour to discover new or collate old facts, etc. by scientific study of a subject, course of critical investigation'. *Concise Oxford Dictionary*, 7th Edition (1982) Oxford University Press, Oxford.

'Research is a scientific process of inquiry and/or experimentation that involves purposeful, systematic, and rigorous collection of data. Analysis and interpretation of the data are then made in order to gain new knowledge or add to existing knowledge. Research has the ultimate aim of developing an organised body of scientific knowledge.' Dempsey, P. A. and Dempsey, A. D. (1986). *The Research Process in Nursing*, Jones and Bartlett, Boston, Mass.; p. 4.

'Research is done to find out. What is happening? How does it work? Which produces better results? Which statement is true? When we want to know something and we are not satisfied with the word of authorities, we do research,' Dixon, B. R., Bouma, G. D. and Atkinson, G. B. J. (1987). *A Handbook of Social Science Research*, Oxford University Press, Oxford; p. 10.

Aim of the exercise To explore some definitions of research.

Planning stage You can do this exercise on your own or in the company of a small group of colleagues, friends or students. Allow yourself plenty of time to complete the exercise and make notes of what you do, as you go. If you work with friends or colleagues, decide whether you will all carry out similar tasks or whether you will divide up the work between you.

Equipment/resources required Notebook, pen and access to a nursing library.

EXERCISE 1.1

What to do

● Read the above definitions and consider the following questions:
  – in what way do these definitions differ from each other if at all?
  – what is meant by the word 'scientific' in any of the definitions?
  – can you be scientific about people?
  – which definition do you prefer and why?
  – does the dictionary definition seem any different to the others? If so, what are the problems of using a dictionary to define words with specific meanings in a particular discipline?
● Read through the following research reports and then consider in what ways these pieces of research support the definitions offered above. If they *do not* in what ways are the above definitions inadequate, if these reports are still to be called research?
  – Firth, H., McIntee, J., McKeown, J. and Britton, P. (1986). Interpersonal Support Amongst Nurses at Work; *Journal of Advanced Nursing*, 11, 273–82.
  – Haase, J. E. (1987). Components of Courage in Chronically Ill Adolescents: A Phenomenological Study; *Advances in Nursing Science*, 9(2), 64–80.
  – Jeffery, R. (1979). Normal Rubbish: deviant patients in casualty departments; *Sociology of Health and Illness*, 1(1), 90–107.

Evaluation Discuss your conclusions with colleagues and with a tutor. Can research be defined easily? What are the problems with definitions in this field? Have your views about research changed as a result of reading research reports?

As another level of evaluation, it is useful, before you finish the activity, to note down:

(a) what you learned from doing the activity;
(b) how you will use what you learned;
(c) how what you have learned relates to what you have read;
(d) what you need to learn next.

2 EXAMPLES OF NURSING RESEARCH

By the end of this section you will have discovered:

● what types of research have been done in nursing.

INFORMATION BOX

Where do you find research reports?

Research is written up in a variety of books, articles and papers. The following list offers some sources of research material:

Books
Magazines and Journals such as:
Nursing Times (Short Reports and Occasional Papers sections),
*Journal of Advanced Nursing,
Nurse Education Today,
Nursing, the add-on Journal,
International Journal of Nursing Studies*
Newspapers
Theses and dissertations
Authors and researchers

Remember that the Inter-Library Loan system, available through most libraries, can arrange for you to see copies of research reports that are not available to you locally. Ask your librarian how this system works and how you can use it.

EXERCISE I.2

Aim of the exercise To explore the range of research that has been done in nursing.

Planning stage You can do this exercise on your own or in the company of a small group of colleagues, friends or students. Allow yourself plenty of time to complete the exercise and make notes of what you do, as you go. If you work with friends or colleagues, decide whether you will all carry out similar tasks or whether you will divide up the work between you.

Equipment/resources required Notebook, pen and access to a nursing library.

What to do

● Read a selection of chapters from the following books to discover some of the *types* of research that have been done in this field:
  – Brooking, J. (ed) (1986). *Psychiatric Nursing Research*; Wiley, Chichester.
  – Clark, J. M. and Hockey, L. (1979). *Research for Nursing: A Guide for the Enquiring Nurse*; HM and M, Aylesbury.
  – Fielding, P. (ed) (1987). *Research in Geriatric Nursing*; Wiley, Chichester.
  – While, A. (ed) (1986). *Research in Preventive Community Nursing Care*; Wiley, Chichester.

● Read the information box on types of nursing research to consider the range of approaches.

● Go to the librarian in your nursing library and ask to see a copy of a nursing research index. Look through this and make a note of some of the research studies that may relate to your own field of interest. Then note down one or two titles of research projects that are *very different to your own areas of interest*. Try to get copies of these reports and read them. Consider the ways in which the various research reports differ from each other and the extent the reports relate to clinical nursing. Were the reports easy to read? Were there difficulties with the terminology used, tables and statistical reports or the author's style of writing?

● What sort of structure did the reports have? Were they clearly laid out with a series of headings and sub headings?

Evaluation Discuss your findings with colleagues and with your tutor. Try to discover if there is a standard format for the layout of research reports. Consider, too, the wide range of nursing research topics, approaches to research and ways of doing research.

- Remember that anyone who has anything important to say will not risk being misunderstood. Has this been true in your experience?

  As another level of evaluation, it is useful, before you finish the activity, to note down:

  (a) what you learned from doing the activity;

  (b) how you will use what you learned;

  (c) how what you have learned relates to what you have read;

  (d) what you need to learn next.

INFORMATION BOX

Types of nursing research

Some research projects are general and broad in approach. Others look at a particular aspect of nursing such as medical nursing. Others consider one topic in nursing like pain and some look at just one specific case or situation. In the diagram below, you can see the progression from the general to the specific. What will your project be: 'broad' in nature or in-depth and very specific?

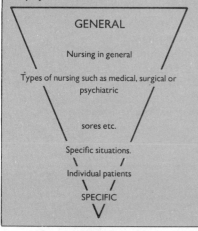

GENERAL

Nursing in general

Types of nursing such as medical, surgical or psychiatric

sores etc.

Specific situations.

Individual patients

SPECIFIC

Another way of considering types of research is to think about the theoretical framework adopted by the researcher. For example, some researchers study their topic from a psychological point of view, some from a sociological standpoint and others from a biological position. Others *combine* various theoretical approaches. In recent years the nursing profession has begun to develop its own body of theories and models. Research is being done to clarify and validate that theoretical base. Here are some examples of nursing research reports which illustrate a particular theoretical position:

- *A psychological study* Davis, B. D. (1983). A Repertory Grid Study of Formal and Informal Aspects of Student Nurse Training; unpublished PhD thesis, University of London.

- *A sociological study* Towell, D. (1975). *Understanding Psychiatric Nursing: A Sociological Study of Modern Psychiatric Practice*, R.C.N., London.

- *A biological study* Hart, J. A. (1985). The Urethral Catheter – A review of its implication in urinary-tract infection; *International Journal of Nursing Studies*, **22**(1), 57–70.

- *A nursing study* Haggerty, L. (1987). An Analysis of Senior US Nursing Students' Immediate Responses to Distressed Patients; *Nursing Times*, **23**(83), 57.

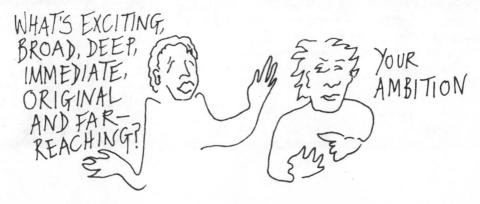

WHAT'S EXCITING, BROAD, DEEP, IMMEDIATE, ORIGINAL AND FAR-REACHING?

YOUR AMBITION

3 STAGES OF THE RESEARCH PROCESS

By the end of this section you will have discovered:

● how to divide up the task of doing research into manageable chunks.

Aim of the exercise To identify the stages of the research process.

Planning stage You can do this exercise on your own or in the company of a small group of colleagues, friends or students. Allow yourself plenty of time to complete the exercise and make notes of what you do, as you go. If you work with friends or colleagues, decide whether you will all carry out similar tasks or whether you will divide up the work between you.

Equipment/resources required Notebook, pen and access to a nursing library.

EXERCISE 1.3

What to do

● Find one nursing research report from each of the following journals. Note differences in style, content, layout and readability in each of the journals:
Nurse Education Today,
Journal of Advanced Nursing,
Nursing Research.
All of these journals use headings and sub-headings in the layout of their research reports and articles. Jot down the heading used in a nursing research report from each of the above journals and look at the similarities and differences between the headings and sub-headings. From this information, try to devise a system of stages that may help to guide you through the process of doing research. Then read the guidelines laid out in the information box, below. To what degree do *your* headings coincide with *ours*?

Evaluation Notice the similarity between the headings used in a written report and the stages of the research process. You can use the headings that you have derived or the headings in our information box for two purposes:
● to guide you in your planning,
● to help you organise the writing up of your project.
As another level of evaluation, it is useful, before you finish the activity, to note down:
(a) what you learned from doing the activity;
(b) how you will use what you learned;
(c) how what you have learned relates to what you have read;
(d) what you need to learn next.

INFORMATION BOX

Stages in the research process

Deciding on the research question	Selecting an appropriate method	This is one way of planning your research. You may find other outlines. The important thing is that you **plan**. You will often find that the stages in the research process overlap in various ways and that you will return to certain stages again and again. Despite this, it is still important to have a very clear initial plan that can serve as a template for your work.
Locating and searching relevant literature	Collecting and storing data	
	Analysing and interpreting data	
Planning the project and preparing a proposal	Drawing conclusions and making recommendations	
Considering ethical issues and getting permission to do the research	Writing and presenting the findings	
Negotiating access to the research site		

4 PLANNING YOUR RESEARCH PROJECT

By the end of this section you will have discovered:

● how to bring structure to your own project and how to plan your work.

Aim of the exercise To explore aspects of your own research project.

Planning stage This exercise should be carried out on your own. Allow yourself plenty of time to complete the exercise and make notes of what you do, as you go.

Equipment/resources required Notebook, pen and access to a nursing library.

EXERCISE 1.4

What to do Make notes about your own research topic under the following headings:

● Deciding on the research question
  – What do you want to find out?
  – Can you write *one sentence* that sums up what you want to do?
This stage of your work is critical. If you can clarify exactly what it is you want to do then the other processes that follow will be much easier. It is worth investing considerable time in clarifying your research question. Discuss this at some length with your tutors and with other people who have had research experience. As you read more and refer to other sources of literature you may want to refine your research question.

● Locating and searching relevant literature
  – Where will you go to find relevant literature?
  – Do you know how to use bibliographies and indexes at your library?
  – Are you familiar with the Inter-Library Loan system?

● Planning the project and preparing a proposal
  – Are there specific guidelines or forms to complete?
  – Have you got someone to oversee your project?
  – Have you seen other people's proposals? If not, have a look at one soon.

● Considering ethical issues and getting permission to do the research
  – Will you be talking to patients? If so, you will probably be required to submit your proposal to an ethics committee. You need to check with your own health authority or department whether or not your project will require ethical approval. This is a critical aspect of your work. You cannot proceed without ethical clearance if this is required.
  – Could anything in your project upset anyone? If you or the person supervising your project has doubts about the sensitive nature of your questions, make sure that you are taking steps to develop skills in handling the responses. Otherwise, leave out any questions that could be upsetting.
  – Do you know how to make a submission to your ethics committee?

● Negotiating access to the research site
  – Who do you approach to get permission to talk to the people you want to interview in your research? It is usual to adopt a 'top–down' approach and ask the most senior person first. You **must** ask permission to interview or talk to people.

● Selecting an appropriate method
  – What methods have been used in this field before?
  – Have they been used successfully?
  – Is it time for a fresh approach?
  – What other approaches are available?

continued

- Collecting and storing data
  - What practical considerations do you need to make with regard to collecting data? Consider, for example, the allocation of time, finding a place to talk to people, expenses to cover postage, travel, typewriting/word processing, and facilities for storing data.

- Analysing and interpreting data
  - Are you familiar with *how* to analyse data? This will be discussed in a later chapter but you must have decided how to analyse data *before you begin to collect it.*

- Drawing conclusions and making recommendations
  - What sort of conclusions do you anticipate drawing? If you can answer this too readily, then you are not remaining open-minded. You are tending to pre-judge the outcome of your research.
  - Who will be interested in your research? For what audience will you be writing?

- Writing and presenting the findings
  - Can you type or use a word processor?
  - Have you got access to such machinery?
  - If not, can you afford to have your work typed by someone else?
  - Will you need to send copies of your report to other people?
  - If so, is there a standard format for such a report?

Evaluation Talk these issues through with colleagues and with your tutor. Note the learning needs that may have arisen as a result of doing this exercise and keep a note of them. At a later stage in your work you may want to return to this exercise again. Your needs and skills will change as you get on with doing your research.

As another level of evaluation, it is useful, before you finish the activity, to note down:

(a) what you learned from doing the activity;

(b) how you will use what you learned;

(c) how what you have learned relates to what you have read;

(d) what you need to learn next.

CONCLUSION

Planning and structuring your project before you start to collect data is vital and will pay huge dividends. It is helpful to sit down with a large pad of paper and make a series of headings and sub-headings, thus dividing up your project into smaller and smaller tasks. This process—which is sometimes known as 'outlining'—can also be done on a personal computer or word processor.

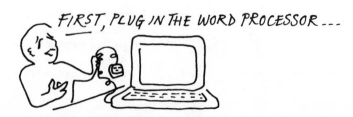

FIRST, PLUG IN THE WORD PROCESSOR...

LEARNING CHECK

If you are a working on your own
- Read through the notes you made while completing the exercises in this chapter and consider the following questions:
  - What new knowledge have I gained?
  - What new skills have I developed?
  - How has my thinking about research changed?
  - What do I need to do now?
- Check that you have made reference cards for any new references that you have found whilst working on the exercises in this chapter.

If you are working in a small group
- Pair off and nominate one of you as A and one of you as B. For five minutes, A talks to B about what has been learned and B listens. This should not be a conversation: B's only role is to listen. After five minutes, roles are reversed and B talks to A about what has been learned and A listens. After the second five minutes, re-form into a group and discuss the experience.

If you are a tutor and/or facilitator
- Use the above 'pairs' exercise with the group you are working with.
- Hold two 'rounds' in which each person in turn says what was liked *least* about doing the activities and what was liked *most* about doing the activities.

2 · PLANNING YOUR RESEARCH PROJECT

WHAT YOU NEED TO READ

Darling, V. H. and Rogers, J. (1986). *Research for Practising Nurses*, Macmillan, London; chapter 2.

Dempsey, P. A. and Dempsey, A. D. (1986). *The Research Process in Nursing*, 2nd Edition, Jones and Bartlett, Boston, Mass.; chapter 3.

Dixon, B. R., Bouma, G. D. and Atkinson, G. B. J. (1987). *A Handbook of Social Science Research: A Comprehensive and Practical Guide for Students*, Oxford University Press, Oxford; chapter 3.

Leedy, P. D. (1985). *Practical Research: Planning and Design*, 3rd Edition, Macmillan, New York; chapters 3, 5 and 6.

AIMS OF THIS CHAPTER

- To help clarify research problems and questions;
- To demonstrate how to write a research proposal;
- To help identify constraints in the research process.

INTRODUCTION

In this chapter we explore the process of planning the research project. We show you how to write a research proposal. Some of the information you need to complete this is covered in later chapters of this book. We suggest that you undertake the exercises here, now. Later on you should return to this chapter and be prepared to modify your proposal.

I CLARIFYING RESEARCH PROBLEMS AND QUESTIONS

By the end of this section you will have discovered:

- how to be specific in the way you identify what your research is about.

EXERCISE 2.1

Aim of the exercise To identify a clear and specific research problem or question.

Planning stage You can do this exercise on your own or in the company of a small group of colleagues, friends or students. Allow yourself plenty of time to complete the exercise and make notes of what you do, as you go. If you work with friends or colleagues, decide whether you will all carry out similar tasks or whether you will divide up the work between you.

Equipment/resources required Notebook, pen and access to a nursing library.

What to do For this exercise, you will be encouraged to use the process known as 'brainstorming'. It is a technique that will be useful in a variety of ways throughout your research work. The information box on page 14 on brainstorming spells out the stages in the process. Read it now.

Using the brainstorming technique, take a large sheet of paper and brainstorm all the sorts of issues in which you are interested as possible fields or aspects of research. A typical list may (or may not) look like this:

- pressure sores
- stress in nurses
- stress in myself
- skill mixes
- interpersonal skills
- counselling skills
- care of the dying
- nursing models: do they work?
- what are nursing models?

As the list above has developed, questions have begun to form. This is the beginning of the process of clarification of a possible research problem or question. Note that the last two items in the list begin to narrow in focus. You will find it helpful to be as specific as you can when you come to framing your research question. We suggest that you work with brainstorming until you can frame your research problem or question *in one sentence*. Some negative and positive examples of research questions include:

- how do nurses care for dying patients?
- are nurses good at interpersonal skills?
- what interpersonal skills do ward sisters identify as being important in dealing with distressed relatives?
- does a nurse's academic ability affect her performance at the clinical level?
- how many patients on ward 'X' have sacral pressure sores of more than 2cm in diameter?
- evaluate the impact of using Orem's Self Care model of nursing in the care of the elderly.
- what factors in nursing are perceived by ward staff as stressful?
- what is the ratio of trained to untrained nursing staff in this hospital?

Look through the list and mark the ones you see as being positive and the ones you see as negative. When you have completed this task, go back to your own work and further refine the question or problem until you are sure that the statement is unambiguous, clear and addresses only a single issue.

Evaluation Check your results with a tutor and discuss the problems of clarifying your own research question or problem. What are the constituents of a good research question? Were the questions or problems clearly stated in the research projects you have read so far? Go back to one of them and try to extract such a question or problem.

As another level of evaluation, it is useful, before you finish the activity, to note down:
(a) what you learned from doing the activity;
(b) how you will use what you learned;
(c) how what you have learned relates to what you have read;
(d) what you need to learn next.

INFORMATION BOX

Brainstorming

This is a method of generating ideas, topics and issues that can be clarified to form a cohesive plan. You will find the technique useful for: clarifying a research question; exploring potential research methods; identifying possible constraints and solutions; identifying new ideas for new projects; problem solving; helping to identify material for an essay or project; uncovering material for a teaching session; sharing a wide range of ideas in a group setting; and developing creativity and intuition.

The technique of brainstorming starts by writing a heading that indicates the broad area that you wish to explore: e.g. *Nursing* or *Counselling* or *Community Care*. Under that heading, and in no particular order, jot down everything that comes to mind when you think about that word. Do not omit anything and do not censor any words, phrases or sentences. Continue this process

until you have either filled the page or you can think of nothing else to write. The process may take anything from five minutes to an hour. The process may also be carried out in a group setting, when one person is elected to act as 'scribe' and then writes down the words called out by other group members.

Now look through the list of words and phrases and strike out any that are not immediately relevant. Be careful, though: you will be surprised how seemingly 'odd' ideas can lead you to a new perspective on the topic. This stage is a period of reflection on the 'free associations' that you have made in the previous stage and links seemingly unconnected ideas.

Finally, place your ideas and associations in an order of priority. In this way you bring structure to your thoughts. You may wish to develop a fairly elaborate system of headings and sub-headings or you may prefer to cluster together

certain related ideas. Either way, you will end the exercise with a wide range of ideas from which to work. Sometimes, you will end up with a huge number of ideas. At other times you will reach just one conclusion, which will usually be your real priority—possibly your research question itself.

Return to this list of ideas and phrases regularly and keep all the paper work involved. In this way you can have a second period of reflection on the material and trace the development of your ideas as they evolve. If the brainstorming procedure does help in the generation of a research question or problem, you will need to spend further time in refining it.

For further details of this method, see Burnard, P. (1988) 'Brainstorming': a practical learning activity in nurse education; *Nurse Education Today*, 8, 354–358.

INFORMATION BOX

Ethical considerations

'Ethics' is concerned with issues of 'right and wrong' and 'good and bad'. In research, ethical questions must be asked at all stages of the process. It is important to continue to ask questions such as:

'Is it right that I am asking people these questions in the process of doing my research?'

'Is what I am doing likely to harm anyone, physically, emotionally or socially?'

'Are my questions *worth* asking? Are they appropriate or important?'

We cannot assume that we have a

right to undertake research or to ask questions of people, without gaining their informed consent. Most district health authorities have ethics committees which ask researchers to submit a copy of their proposal. You must be clear about the ethical requirements and procedures in your district before you proceed beyond the planning stage. Many district ethics committees have a standard form to be submitted with the research proposal. The committee may also ask to interview you about your proposal. It is important not to

overlook ethical issues when planning research, and to discuss any proposals that you have— particularly if they involve asking for patients' cooperation—with a colleague, tutor or lecturer.

Useful references on this topic are:
– Burnard, P. and Chapman, C. (1988) *Professional and Ethical Issues in Nursing: The Code of Professional Conduct*; Wiley, Chichester.
– RCN (1977) *Ethics Related to Research in Nursing*; Royal College of Nursing, London.

2 WRITING A RESEARCH PROPOSAL

By the end of this section you will have discovered:

● how to write a research proposal.

A research proposal is a detailed statement of what you intend to do, why you want to do it and how you will go about it. It shows your ability to carry through the project and whether the design and methods you have selected are appropriate to the problem you have selected. The process of drawing up a research proposal can help you to clarify your thoughts and methods. It is also necessary to allow other people to examine your project and its methods. This is particularly true of those projects that require clearance from ethics committees.

Writing a research proposal often takes a considerable amount of time. You may have to rough out various drafts and the people to whom you submit the proposal may ask you to make changes. Don't be put off by this. Do not *refuse* to make changes. You run the risk of supervision or support being withdrawn if you do.

In the information box below on guidelines you will find a structured outline for producing a research proposal. Note that this is only one way of drawing up such a document. Your school, college, awarding body or local authority may have another format. But if so, the basic structure of the proposal will always be similar to the one in the information box.

INFORMATION BOX

Guidelines for a research proposal

The research proposal you produce should be written in the following order:

Title of the project

Name and designation of the researcher

Supervisor

Department

Statement of the problem

Aims and objectives of the project

Rationale for doing the research

Course of study being undertaken (if applicable)

Brief review of the relevant literature

Research methods

Methods of data analysis

Preparation of report

Ethical considerations

Costs involved

Other considerations not covered above

Curriculum Vitae of researcher.

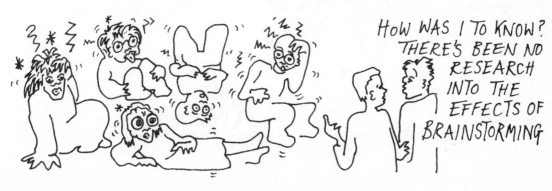

HOW WAS I TO KNOW? THERE'S BEEN NO RESEARCH INTO THE EFFECTS OF BRAINSTORMING

Aim of the exercise To draw up a research proposal.

Planning stage You can do this exercise on your own or in the company of a small group of colleagues, friends or students. Allow yourself plenty of time to complete the exercise and make notes of what you do, as you go. If you work with friends or colleagues, decide whether you will all carry out similar tasks or whether you will divide up the work between you.

Equipment/resources required Notebook, pen and access to a nursing library.

EXERCISE 2.2

What to do Read through the information box *Guidelines for a research proposal* and make notes about your own research under those headings. Continue to refine your proposal until you are sure it is clear, detailed and complete.

Evaluation Show your proposal to a tutor and take note of any modifications that are suggested. After you have written the proposal, ask yourself the following questions:

- Is the proposal realistic? Have I the necessary skills to undertake this piece of research? Have I the time to carry it through? Do I know how to complete the various stages?
- Is the proposal clear? Have I used simple, unambiguous language and avoided jargon? Always explain technical terms, especially if the proposal is going to be read by those unfamiliar with research. Remember that your proposal may need further amendments as you develop your thoughts and ideas.
- Have I covered each aspect of the proposal thoroughly?
- Does the proposal state exactly what I want to do and how I intend to do it?
- Can I anticipate any sections of the proposal which may cause others to be concerned or to ask questions? Always be prepared for questions from other people, especially from supervisors and ethics committees.

As another level of evaluation, it is useful, before you finish the activity, to note down:
(a) what you learned from doing the activity;
(b) how you will use what you learned;
(c) how what you have learned relates to what you have read;
(d) what you need to learn next.

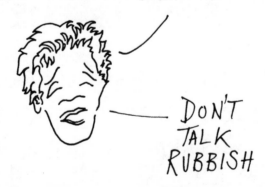

INTRODUCE PREVENTATIVE INTERVENTIONAL CAPACITY INTO VALUE-FREE SPEECH

DON'T TALK RUBBISH

INFORMATION BOX

Writing a Curriculum Vitae

You will need a Curriculum Vitae (CV) on many occasions such as when you are preparing a research proposal. The CV should be typed and should set out your life history to date. Your CV allows the reader an opportunity to assess your suitability for undertaking the research. A CV also shows what you have studied and the work that you have done. It is worth investing time in the preparation of a CV and it is a good idea to keep copies of it.

A sample Curriculum Vitae appears on pages 76–8.

It is usual to divide a CV into sections for clarity. A typical CV would include the following headings:

Name

Home address

Home telephone number

Nationality

Marital status

Age

Date of birth

Occupation

Work address

Work phone number

Schools and colleges attended (with dates)

Examinations passed (with grades and dates)

Other educational achievements (awards, grants, scholarships etc)

Professional training (places, dates, qualifications obtained)

Posts held (most recent first)

Present post

Brief outline of responsibilities in present post

Salary scale and point on the scale

Professional courses attended

Publications and/or previous research

Hobbies and interests

Other details (such as ability to type and other skills not entered elsewhere).

If you work with a computer or word processor, it is worth keeping a copy of your CV on disk and updating as your circumstances change.

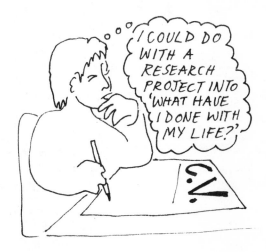

I COULD DO WITH A RESEARCH PROJECT INTO 'WHAT HAVE I DONE WITH MY LIFE?'

3 IDENTIFYING CONSTRAINTS

By the end of this section you will have discovered:

● what constraints are likely to effect your research.

EXERCISE 2.3

Aim of the exercise To explore constraints as they apply to your project.

Planning stage You can do this exercise on your own or in the company of a small group of colleagues, friends or students. Allow yourself plenty of time to complete the exercise and make notes of what you do, as you go. If you work with friends or colleagues, decide whether you will all carry out similar tasks or you will divide up the work between you.

Equipment/resources required Notebook, pen and access to a nursing library.

What to do Sit on your own and write down the headings in the table. The table will allow you to identify any snags in your project and anything that may stand in the way of completing it. In the second column of the table, you are encouraged to use a problem-solving approach to find ways of dealing with the constraints that you have identified. You are then asked to plan action to help overcome any constraints. The process of doing the exercise will make the next stages of your project easier.

Possible constraint	Suggestions for how constraint may be managed	Action
Brainstorm all possible constraints, here. They may include such things as ● other people's attitudes ● time factors ● financial limitations ● ethical issues ● lack of knowledge about research.	Identify ideas for managing each constraint. Some may be insurmountable but at least you will be prepared and you will be better able to plan what you need to do next.	Write in here *realistic* things to be done and how you will do them.

Table for exploring possible constraints in your research project.

Evaluation What constraints did you identify? If you identified large constraints or a high number you may have to rethink part of your project and reduce your expectations. Discuss your findings with your colleagues and with a tutor and ask them to state what *they* think may be the constraints in *your* project. Be prepared to accept criticism and be prepared to alter your strategy.

At this stage, you may want to consider a pilot study, which is a small project to allow you to discover whether or not your plan works. The pilot study can be an ideal way of uncovering problems. Once discovered, these issues can be considered and your plan can be modified.

As another level of evaluation, it is useful, before you finish the activity, to note down:
(a) what you learned from doing the activity;
(b) how you will use what you learned;
(c) how what you have learned relates to what you have read;
(d) what you need to learn next.

CONCLUSION

By now you should have prepared your proposal and be reasonably confident that you can carry out the research. The time that you spend in planning will not be wasted. It is preferable to iron out as many problems at this stage as possible rather than make substantial changes during the research itself.

LEARNING CHECK

If you are a working on your own
● Read through the notes you made while completing the exercises in this chapter and consider the following questions:
  – What new knowledge have I gained?
  – What new skills have I developed?
  – How has my thinking about research changed?
  – What do I need to do now?
● Check that you have made reference cards for any new references that you have found whilst working on the exercises in this chapter.

If you are working in a small group
● Pair off and nominate one of you as A and one of you as B. For five minutes, A talks to B about what has been learned and B listens. This should not be a conversation: B's only role is to listen. After five minutes, roles are reversed and B talks to A about what has been learned and A listens. After the second five minutes, re-form into a group and discuss the experience.

If you are a tutor and/or facilitator
● Use the above 'pairs' exercise with the group you are working with.
● Hold two 'rounds' in which each person in turn says what was liked *least* about doing the activities and what was liked *most* about doing the activities.

3 · SEARCHING THE LITERATURE

WHAT YOU NEED TO READ

Bell, J. (1987). *Doing Your Research Project: A Guide for First-Time Researchers in Education and Social Science*, Open University Press, Milton Keynes; chapters 3 and 4.

Cormack, D. F. S. (ed) (1984). *The Research Process in Nursing*, Blackwell, Oxford; chapters 7 and 20.

Haywood, P. and Wragg, E. C. (1982). *Evaluating the Literature*, Rediguide 2, Guides in Educational Research, Nottingham University, Nottingham.

Macleod Clark, J. and Stodulski, A. H. (1978). How to Find Out: A Guide to Searching the Nursing Literature, *Nursing Times*, 74, 6, 21–23.

Pollock, L. (1984). Six Steps to a Successful Literature Search, *Nursing Times*, 80, **44**, 40–43.

AIMS OF THIS CHAPTER

- To explore literature resources;
- To discuss how to conduct a literature search;
- To consider how to review literature critically;
- To encourage writing a literature review.

INTRODUCTION

This chapter focuses on the skills you will need to search for literature relevant to your project. A systematic search of the work already carried out in your field is necessary so that you know what has been done.

When you have completed the search, you will be able to:

- summarise the previous research to help you formulate your own ideas;
- have a better idea about what approaches and methods other researchers have used and make an informed choice about different procedures;
- identify important omissions in the work that has already been completed and design your study so that you are adding to the established body of knowledge.

You may wish to follow up published material by contacting the authors to clarify issues raised in their work or to discuss possible lines of inquiry. It is worth noting that you must continue to search the literature throughout all the stages of the research process. Your field of study is constantly changing. You must keep up to date!

I EXPLORING THE LITERATURE RESOURCES

By the end of this section you will have discovered:

● where to find information about previous work.

Aim of the exercise To identify literature resources.

Planning stage You can do this exercise on your own or in the company of a small group of colleagues, friends or students. Allow yourself plenty of time to complete the exercise and make notes of what you do, as you go. If you work with friends or colleagues, decide whether you will all carry out similar tasks or whether you will divide up the work between you.

Equipment/resources required Notebook, pen and access to a nursing library.

EXERCISE 3.1

What to do Draw three concentric circles on a page like the example here. The inner circle represents literature that is *immediately* available, such as your own books. The middle circle represents literature that is available within easy reach—at the school of nursing library for example. The outer circle represents literature that is available with some effort like the Inter-Library Loan scheme. Personalise the diagram so that it becomes a source of reference for you when you do your literature searching. Add to it as you discover new sources of information and keep it with you throughout your research project. Also, keep a list of the libraries and resource centres that you have visited and the sections in those departments that you have explored. In this way, you become more systematic in your search and avoid unnecessary repetition.

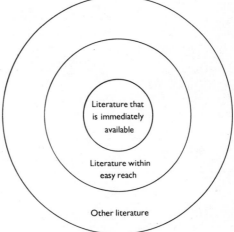

Evaluation Go through the information contained in the three circles and identify which sources you are using at present. Write a list of those sources about which you want more information. Also list the sources that you will use in the coming weeks. Do any of the sources *charge* for their services? If so, have you budgeted for this? Are any of the sources likely to take time to respond to your request? Did you account for this in your planning? If not, would it be better to seek this information from another source? Do you really need this information? Is it *vital* to your project? If you have doubts about this, talk to your supervisor. A great deal of time can be lost searching out obscure material that only partly relates to the project.

As another level of evaluation, it is useful, before you finish the activity, to note down:

(a) what you learned from doing the activity;
(b) how you will use what you learned;
(c) how what you have learned relates to what you have read;
(d) what you need to learn next.

2 FINDING AND SUMMARISING RELEVANT LITERATURE

By the end of this section you will have discovered:

- how to find literature and information as part of your research project;
- how to keep records of the literature you find.

INFORMATION BOX

Guidelines for evaluating research reports

As you go through the literature, you will find reports of other people's research. The following guidelines will help you ask questions about that research and allow you to establish your ideas about problems, methods and analytical techniques in your own research project.

The research problem
is it clearly stated?
is it easily researched?
does it relate directly to nursing?

The literature review
is it relevant to the topic?
is it comprehensive?
how current are the sources of literature?
is the referencing method used correctly?
is the review laid out logically?
is a summary placed at the end of the review that spells out implications for the present study?

Design of the study
is there a statement of the overall design?
is there a discussion about the theoretical framework?
if hypotheses are offered, are they clearly stated?
is there a clear description of what the researcher planned to do, what the researcher did and how the researcher did it?
are relevant technical terms defined clearly?

Data collection
is the method described clearly?
does the researcher justify the use of the method?
is the sample discussed in terms of relevance and size?
are instruments used clearly described?
are reliability and validity addressed? (See Chapter 6.)
is there a clear description of what the researcher did when the data was collected?

Data analysis
are the methods appropriate for the data?
are those methods clearly described?
is the presentation of findings clearly laid out?
is there adequate discussion of results?

Conclusions and recommendations
are they justified?
are they linked sufficiently with the original purpose?
are the recommendations practical?
are implications for further research discussed?
are the limitations of the study discussed?

INFORMATION BOX

Reviewing other literature

Apart from reviewing research reports, you will want to read other sorts of literature such as books, biographies, policy documents, and official reports. As you read, consider whether or not arguments are expressed clearly and if they are substantiated by reference to research or rational argument. Are the assumptions underlying the argument spelt out and are the limitations of a particular argument identified? You should decide whether the author adopts a particular position which blocks other possibilities. Consider also whether the arguments are relevant to your subject area and if they flow logically. Another thing to think about is whether technical terms are explained properly.

These are not the only issues which you should explore when reading literature but they will help you to evaluate what you read and to become more critical.

EXERCISE 3.2

Aim of the exercise To find a specific piece of information from a library.

Planning stage Prepare to go to a library which contains a reasonable selection of books and journals on nursing. Allow yourself plenty of time to complete the exercise and make notes of what you do, as you go.

Equipment/resources required Notebook, pen, access to a nursing library, transport.

What to do Go to the library and ask the librarian to explain the cataloguing system to you. Find the following publications or articles and make notes of how and where you found them. Note the library cataloguing number on the spine of the book. (This information will be important for the next exercise.)

– Field, P. A. and Morse, J. M. (1985). *Nursing Research: The Application of Qualitative Approaches*; Croom Helm, London.
– Fielding, R. G. and Llewelyn, S. P. (1987). Communication training in nursing may damage your health and enthusiasm; some warnings; *Journal of Advanced Nursing*, **12**, 281–290.

Evaluation What problems did you have in using the cataloguing system? What was the name of the cataloguing system? Did you ask the librarian to find the publications for you? If you did, will you know your way around the library next time? How did you record the information about where the publications were located?

As another level of evaluation, it is useful, before you finish the activity, to note down:
(a) what you learned from doing the activity;
(b) how you will use what you learned;
(c) how what you have learned relates to what you have read;
(d) what you need to learn next.

INFORMATION BOX

Abstracts

Do not be too narrow in your search for relevant literature. Consider abstracts of papers in the social, biological and behavioural sciences, as well as those in nursing. Indexes of abstracts include:

Applied Social Science Index and Abstracts (ASSIA)
Current Contents
Psychological Abstracts
Social Science Citation Index (SSCI).

Also think about the growing number of *computerised* abstracting services. Your local library may be able to organise a computer search of the literature. However such searches can be costly and may produce many unwanted references. You can also get lists of abstracts on disk, from various suppliers.

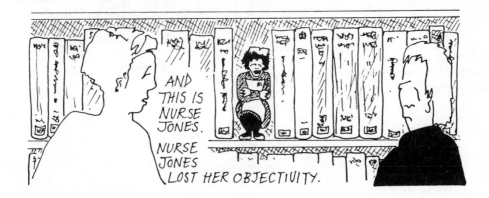

23

3 KEEPING A CARD REFERENCE SYSTEM

By the end of this section you will have discovered:

● how to keep a record of what you read;
● how to organise these records.

Aims of the exercise To demonstrate how you can make useful notes from what you read, and how to organise these notes.

Planning stage You will need access to your library again. Allow yourself plenty of time to complete the exercise and make notes of what you do, as you go.

Equipment required Index cards, a box for filing the cards, a pen.

EXERCISE 3.3

What to do Go to your library and find the article by Fielding and Llewelyn (1987) and the book by Field and Morse (1985) which were listed in the previous exercise. Answer the following questions:

● what factors hamper the development of communications training in the Fielding and Llewelyn (1987) paper?
● what is the purpose of qualitative research according to Field and Morse (1985)?

Once you have answered the questions you will need to make an accurate record of what the authors have said, in support of your answers. Details about the sources of your literature are required so that your project can be written and referenced accurately. We recommend that you use the following system.

Prepare your index cards as shown in the diagram below. You can adapt the layout to suit your own needs but once you have settled on a format, stick to it. Always have index cards with you, so that when you find a new and relevant reference you can make notes about it. Make sure that your referencing system is thorough.

```
AUTHOR    DATE    (for books)
                  TITLE
                  EDITION
                  PUBLISHER
                  PLACE OF PUBLICATION

                  (for journal articles)
                  TITLE
                  VOLUME NUMBER
                  EDITION NUMBER
                  PAGE NUMBERS

Summary of relevant points.
(Direct quotes must have page numbers.)
```

Llewelyn, S.P. and Trent, R.T. 1987 Nursing in the Community
British Psychological Society
Methuen
London

Useful chapter on sex and the patient (pp. 83-97). Discussion of caring for the elderly person in the community.
Describes the importance of the relationships between nurses and patients in the community.
'... how people behave and feel in sickness and distress can only really be understood if you also know about their current life situations and what their background is. Different expectations, values, religious beliefs and types of family support mean that things which may only be a minor inconvenience for one person may create a very serious problem for someone else.' (p4)

An example of an index card layout and how it would appear when completed.

continued

Evaluation You may have been tempted to use the authors' words to answer the questions, but it is better to write your own synopsis. Use quotations sparingly and remember to put them in inverted commas and record the precise page number. Keep your cards in alphabetical order in a plastic box. It is useful to cross-reference your cards or put them in sections under subject headings.

As another level of evaluation, it is useful, before you finish the activity, to note down:

(a) what you learned from doing the activity;
(b) how you will use what you learned;
(c) how what you have learned relates to what you have read;
(d) what you need to learn next.

INFORMATION BOX

Computer records

Many people now use personal computers and word processors. Programs are available which simulate a card-index system. These programs allow you to design your own formats for cards and many allow you to find all the cards that relate to one subject or all the cards that refer to a particular author. These programs are called databases and vary in their complexity. It is important to ask for advice about which one would best suit your needs. If a computer index is used it is important that copies of the index are kept and updated at regular intervals. If you do not make back-up copies and there is a power cut while you are using your computer, you stand to lose the whole of your reference system!

4 CRITICALLY REVIEWING THE LITERATURE

By the end of this section you will have discovered:

● how to review critically what you read.

EXERCISE 3.4

Aim of the exercise To explore styles of critical literature reviewing.

Planning stage Negotiate access to a library that will be able to supply you with the articles referred to below. Allow time for reading and writing comments.

Equipment/resources required Notebook, pen, access to a nursing library, transport.

What to do Read the literature review sections of the following two articles. Compare the two styles of reviewing and note how each author uses references to other work. Note whether or not they are *critical* of other people's work. It is important that reviews of the literature do not become lists of other research or theories.

As you read, look to see if the author breaks the review up into sections and if the methodology of previous research is questioned. Does the author challenge the assumptions that previous writers make? Do you understand the points that are made? Also think about whether the review is interesting or balanced.

Keep asking questions about what you are reading. Challenge what is written and look for explanations of the arguments. This is the process of *critical evaluation*. Note, however, that to be 'critical' is not just picking holes in the work. It is also discriminating between the 'good' and 'bad' parts of the work.

The two articles for consideration are:
– Goodman, C. (1986). Research on the Informal Carer. A Selected Literature Review; *Journal of Advanced Nursing*, 11, 705–712.

continued

25

– McCloskey, J. C. (1981). The Effects of Nursing Education on Job Effectiveness: An Overview of the Literature; *Research in Nursing and Health*, 4, 355–373.

Complete an index card for each of these articles and make notes about the content of the two papers. In this way you will reinforce the habit of keeping notes of your reading.

Evaluation Read through your notes, consider your summaries and then ask a colleague to read one of the papers and discuss your individual views. Note how different people's perceptions of the same paper can vary considerably!

As another level of evaluation, it is useful, before you finish the activity, to note down:

(a) what you learned from doing the activity;
(b) how you will use what you learned;
(c) how what you have learned relates to what you have read;
(d) what you need to learn next.

5 WRITING A LITERATURE REVIEW

By the end of this section you will have discovered:

● how to write your own literature review.

EXERCISE 3.5

Aim of the exercise To undertake a short literature review.

Planning stage Identify a topic of your choice. Identify the literature resources relevant to your chosen area. Arrange access to your local library.

Equipment/resources required Index cards and box, pen, transport.

What to do Go to your library and find ten articles or books related to your chosen subject. Make a summary of each of these on the index cards. Write a critical review of the ten articles of not more than 500–1000 words.

Evaluation Choose one of the following options:

● show the review to your tutor or supervisor;
● ask friends or colleagues to read and comment on it;
● share the review with a group of colleagues who have also undertaken the exercise.

As another level of evaluation, it is useful, before you finish the activity, to note down:

(a) what you learned from doing the activity;
(b) how you will use what you learned;
(c) how what you have learned relates to what you have read;
(d) what you need to learn next.

CONCLUSION

You should now be able to collect information relating to your area of interest and record the details of that information on index cards. You should also be developing an awareness of how to read and write a critical literature review. The skills learnt in this stage of the research process will be required throughout the development of your project.

LEARNING CHECK

If you are a working on your own

- Read through the notes you have made while completing the exercises in this chapter and consider the following questions:
    - What new knowledge have I gained?
    - What new skills have I developed?
    - How has my thinking about research changed?
    - What do I need to do now?
- Check that you have completed index cards for any new references that you have found whilst working on the exercises in this chapter.

If you are working in a small group

- Pair off and nominate one of you as A and one of you as B. For five minutes, A talks to B about what has been learned and B listens. This should not be a conversation: B's only role is to listen. After five minutes, roles are reversed and B talks to A about what has been learned and A listens. After the second five minutes, re-form into a group and discuss the experience.

If you are a tutor and/or facilitator

- Use the above 'pairs' exercise with the group you are working with.
- Hold two 'rounds' in which each person in turn says what was liked *least* about doing the activities and what was liked *most* about doing the activities.

4 • APPROACHES TO RESEARCH METHODOLOGY

WHAT YOU NEED TO READ

Cormack, D. F. S. (ed) (1984). *The Research Process in Nursing*, Blackwell, Oxford.

Dixon, B. R., Bouma, G. D. and Atkinson, G. B. J. (1987). *A Handbook of Social Science Research: A Comprehensive and Practical Guide for Students*, Oxford University Press, Oxford.

Field, P. A. and Morse, J. M. (1985). *Nursing Research: The Application of Qualitative Approaches*, Croom Helm, London.

Morgan, G. and Smircich, L. (1980). The Case for Qualitative Research, *Academy of Management Review*, 5, 4, 491–500.

Reason, P. and Rowan, J. (eds) (1981). *Human Inquiry: A Sourcebook of New Paradigm Research*, Wiley, Chichester; chapters 1 and 2.

Skevington, S. (ed) (1984). *Understanding Nurses: The Social Psychology of Nursing*, Wiley, Chichester.

AIMS OF THIS CHAPTER

- To list the distinguishing characteristics of quantitative and qualitative methods of research;
- To discriminate between descriptive and experimental research;
- To identify the problems associated with subjectivity and objectivity;
- To help you consider which approach is most appropriate for your research.

INTRODUCTION

There are different approaches to research. Sometimes it is useful to count and categorise things but at other times it is better to find out how people perceive matters. This chapter explores some differences between various approaches to research. The temptation to polarise thinking into approaches being 'either/or' is a strong one. We hope that in looking at the different concepts involved in this chapter you will see the various approaches as *complementary* rather than competitive.

I THE DIFFERENCES BETWEEN QUANTITATIVE AND QUALITATIVE RESEARCH

By the end of this section you will have discovered:

- what the two words mean;
- how quantitative and qualitative research can be distinguished;
- some examples of quantitative and qualitative research.

EXERCISE 4.1

Aim of the exercise To define the words 'quantitative' and 'qualitative'.

Planning stage This exercise can be carried out either by an individual or by a group of people. Allow yourself plenty of time to complete the exercise and make notes of what you do. If you work with friends or colleagues, decide whether you will all carry out similar tasks or whether you will divide up the work between you.

Equipment/resources required Notebook, pen and access to a nursing library.

What to do Find three of the references referred to in the *What you need to read* box and look at how the writers use the words 'quantitative' and 'qualitative'. Then look up those words in a dictionary and compare the definitions to the ways the words were used in the research literature.

Evaluation Discuss the various definitions of the two approaches and consider how you may draw out characteristics that distinguish the two approaches from one another.

As another level of evaluation, it is useful, before you finish the activity, to note down:

(a) what you learned from doing the activity;
(b) how you will use what you learned;
(c) how what you have learned relates to what you have read;
(d) what you need to learn next.

EXERCISE 4.2

Aim of the exercise To identify the characteristics that differentiate quantitative and qualitative approaches to research.

Planning stages Prepare to go to a library which contains a reasonable selection of books on research. This activity can be carried out alone or in a small group. Allow yourself plenty of time to complete the exercise and make notes of what you do. If you work with friends or colleagues, decide whether you will all carry out similar tasks or whether you will divide up the work between you.

Equipment/resources required Notebook, pen and access to a nursing library.

What to do Read books on research and complete a grid like that shown below. The grid offers you certain criteria for distinguishing the practical differences between the two approaches. It also asks you to find three examples of each type of research from the literature.

	Quantitative research	Qualitative research
Purpose of the research		
Sample size		
Data collection methods		
Data analysis methods		
Method of presenting findings		
Three examples from the nursing literature		

Grid for comparing quantitative and qualitative research.

Evaluation Discuss these lists with a colleague or with the group with which you are working. Compare what others say with your own work. Is it possible to make a clear distinction between the two? What types of research problems lend themselves to the different approaches? Have any nursing research studies used both approaches?

As another level of evaluation, it is useful, before you finish the activity, to note down:

(a) what you learned from doing the activity;
(b) how you will use what you learned;
(c) how what you have learned relates to what you have read;
(d) what you need to learn next.

2 DESCRIPTIVE AND EXPERIMENTAL RESEARCH

By the end of this section you will have discovered:

● the differences between descriptive and experimental research.

Aim of the exercise To identify the differences between descriptive and experimental research.

Planning stage This exercise can be carried out by an individual or by a group. Allow yourself plenty of time to complete the exercise and make notes of what you do. If you work with friends or colleagues, decide whether you will all carry out similar tasks or whether you will divide up the work between you.

Equipment/resources required Notebook, pen and access to a nursing library.

EXERCISE 4.3

What to do Read the following four research reports which illustrate some different approaches to doing research.

– Bogdan, R., Brown, M. A. and Foster, S. B. (1982). Be Honest But Not Cruel: Staff/Patient Communication on a Neonatal Unit; *Human Organisation*, 41, 1, 6–16.
– Burnard, P. and Morrison, P. (1988). Nurses' Perceptions of Their Interpersonal Skills: a Descriptive Study Using Six Category Intervention Analysis; *Nurse Education Today*, 8, 266–272.
– Hayward, J. (1975). *Information: A Prescription Against Pain*; RCN, London.
– Luker, K. A. (1982). *Evaluating Health Visiting Practice*; RCN, London.

Now answer the following questions:

● what methods did each study use?
● what sort of information was collected?
● how was the data analysed?
● what generalisations were made by the researchers?

Now read the next information box on descriptive and experimental research. Which type of approach was used in the four studies?

Evaluation Check your decisions with a colleague or a tutor.

As another level of evaluation, it is useful, before you finish the activity, to note down:

(a) what you learned from doing the activity;
(b) how you will use what you learned;
(c) how what you have learned relates to what you have read;
(d) what you need to learn next.

INFORMATION BOX
Descriptive and experimental research

The many differences between descriptive and experimental research often depend on individual attitudes. For example, a person drawn to *experimental* research may believe that there are many similarities between people or that behaviour is causally determined. He/she may then develop a hypothesis and experimentally prove, or disprove, it. A person drawn to *descriptive* research may describe a place, situation or environment, believing that what is important in research is to note different perceptions of the world.

Our beliefs about the nature of the world and of the people that inhabit it will affect the sorts of questions we ask; the way we approach planning our research; the sorts of research methods we use; the way we interpret the data we collect and the conclusions we draw from our findings.

Some distinctions can be made between the two approaches:

Descriptive research merely describes something, whereas experimental research tests an hypothesis;

Researchers can control variables in experimental research but cannot do this with descriptive research;

Descriptive research is subjective, but experimental research is objective;

Experimental research can lead to predictions, but descriptive research cannot do this.

4 SUBJECTIVITY AND OBJECTIVITY IN RESEARCH

By the end of this section you will have discovered:

● some of the differences between subjectivity and objectivity;
● some of the problems associated with these two concepts.

EXERCISE 4.4

Aim of the exercise To explore the problems of subjectivity and objectivity.

Planning stage The exercise needs to be carried out with a small group of friends or colleagues. Allow yourself plenty of time to complete the exercise and make notes of what you do. Decide whether you will all carry out similar tasks or whether you will divide up the work between you.

Equipment/resources required Notebook, pen and access to a nursing library.

What to do Look up the words 'subjectivity' and 'objectivity' in a dictionary. Then look at some books on research and read about how researchers have battled with the notions of subjectivity and objectivity. With your colleagues, sit and write individual descriptions of the room you are in at present. Write about one page. Read out your reports and decide whose description was the most accurate, most objective and most interesting. Whose was the most different to all the others?

Now hold a discussion on the topic of subjectivity and objectivity and try to answer the following questions:

● how can you attempt to be objective in research?
● do you need to be?
● if so, why?
● is objectivity possible?
● is there a place in research for the subjective report?
● if so, what is that place?

Evaluation Read through a research report and note the degree to which the researcher has addressed the issue of objectivity. A useful paper, here, is:
– LeCompte, M. D. and Goetz, J. P. (1982). Problems of Reliability and Validity in Ethnographic Research; *Review of Educational Research*, 52, 1, 31–60.

As another level of evaluation, it is useful, before you finish the activity, to note down:
(a) what you learned from doing the activity;
(b) how you will use what you learned;
(c) how what you have learned relates to what you have read;
(d) what you need to learn next.

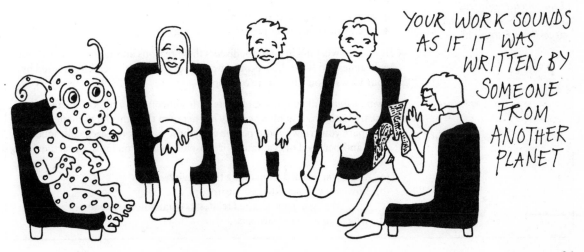

YOUR WORK SOUNDS AS IF IT WAS WRITTEN BY SOMEONE FROM ANOTHER PLANET

5 SELECTING OR BLENDING THE APPROACHES

As you have worked through this chapter you will have begun to address some of the complexities and ambiguities of research. In order to make decisions about which approach you should use, you will have to become clear about your own beliefs about human beings and about how you view the world. You cannot detach yourself so that you are completely objective. For a further discussion of this issue, read the first two chapters of:

– Reason, P. and Rowan, J. (eds) (1981). *Human Inquiry: A Sourcebook of New Paradigm Research*; Wiley, Chichester.

By the end of this section you will have discovered:

● more about yourself;
● more about how your own beliefs influence the way you do research.

Aim of the exercise To explore individual beliefs about research.

Planning stage This activity can be carried out alone or with a group of other people. Allow yourself plenty of time to complete the exercise and make notes of what you do. If you work with friends or colleagues, decide whether you will all carry out similar tasks or whether you will divide up the work between you.

Equipment/resources required Notebook, pen and access to a nursing library.

EXERCISE 4.5

What to do Write some notes on your beliefs about people. Do you believe, for example, that a person's personality is shaped by society or that a person is born with a certain personality? Or do you think that people can change themselves in fundamental ways? Whatever you think about people just jot down some notes on your beliefs. If you are working in a group, discuss your notes with your colleagues. If alone, go through the paper and turn each of your statements into a question. If you have written: 'People are corrupted by society', ask the question 'Are people corrupted by society?' In this way, you begin to think critically about your own beliefs and assumptions. Try to argue *against* each of the questions.

Now write out a short report on what you believe to be the functions and uses of research. Some of the things you may want to consider include the following:

● to add to the body of knowledge;
● to develop a greater understanding of people and the world;
● to attempt to predict the future;
● to contribute to other people's well-being.

If you are working in a group, discuss these reasons and functions with your colleagues. To what degree are your reasons for doing research coloured by your views about the nature of people?

Evaluation Talk about your beliefs with someone who has completed a research project. Ask him/her how his/her own thoughts have changed. Compare your views about people with those of your research colleague.

As another level of evaluation, it is useful, before you finish the activity, to note down:
(a) what you learned from doing the activity;
(b) how you will use what you learned;
(c) how what you have learned relates to what you have read;
(d) what you need to learn next.

CONCLUSION

Until you have thought about some of the basic questions about people and research you have not developed the ability to be critical. Research has the interesting effect of challenging all our cherished beliefs and values.

LEARNING CHECK

If you are a working on your own
- Read through the notes you made while completing the exercises in this chapter and consider the following questions:
  - What new knowledge have I gained?
  - What new skills have I developed?
  - How has my thinking about research changed?
  - What do I need to do now?
- Check that you have made reference cards for any new references that you have found whilst working on the exercises in this chapter.

If you are working in a small group
- Pair off and nominate one of you as A and one of you as B. For five minutes, A talks to B about what has been learned and B listens. This should not be a conversation: B's only role is to listen. After five minutes, roles are reversed and B talks to A about what has been learned and A listens. After the second five minutes, re-form into a group and discuss the experience.

If you are a tutor and/or facilitator
- Use the above 'pairs' exercise with the group you are working with.
- Hold two 'rounds' in which each person in turn says what was liked *least* about doing the activities and what was liked *most* about doing the activities.

5 · CHOOSING A RESEARCH METHOD

WHAT YOU NEED TO READ

Dixon, B. R., Bouma, G. D. and Atkinson, G. B. J. (1987). *A Handbook of Social Science Research: A Comprehensive and Practical Guide for Students*, Oxford University Press, Oxford; chapter 6.

Long, A. F. (1984). *Research into Health and Illness: Issues in Design, Analysis and Practice*, Gower, Aldershot.

Omery, A. (1983). Phenomenology: A Method for Nursing Research, *Advances in Nursing Science*, 5, 2, 49–63.

Reason, P. and Rowan, J. (eds) (1981). *Human Inquiry: A Sourcebook of New Paradigm Research*, Wiley, Chichester; Introduction.

AIMS OF THIS CHAPTER

- To point out issues that help you to make decisions about methods;
- To identify how to find out about the range of methods available in order to make an informed decision;
- To establish the method of data collection you will use in your project;
- To clarify how your data is going to be analysed after collection.

INTRODUCTION

By now you will have established your research question and will be considering ways of collecting data that will help you answer that question. The next issue is that of deciding which is the most effective way of collecting information. Before you go ahead and collect research data you need to be clear about the method you are going to use to collect it. By the end of this chapter you will be clearer about what sort of method you want to choose. Much will depend, of course, on what you want to find out.

It is vital that you understand how you will process your data when you have collected it. Many researchers can tell you about people who have collected masses of data who then don't know what to do with it. In planning your method of data collection, you must select your method of analysis.

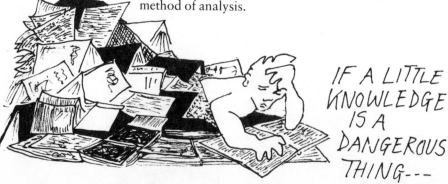

IF A LITTLE KNOWLEDGE IS A DANGEROUS THING---

INFORMATION BOX

The concept of research design

The term 'research design' is sometimes used for a particular approach to doing research. The three designs commonly used are survey, experiment and case study. *A survey* is the systematic gathering of information. The purpose is to identify general trends or patterns in data. Examples of surveys are:

nurses' attitudes to smoking;

the number of enrolled nurses at a particular hospital during a particular period;

the incidence of a specific illness in different parts of the country.

The experiment sets out to test an hypothesis. Experimental research tries to establish causal links between a number of factors. Examples include:

the effect of the provision of information on the rate of recovery from illness;

the effectiveness of a specific drug in treating a particular disorder.

The case study is a detailed account of a small number of examples of a particular experience, event or situation. The aim of the case study approach is to 'paint a picture', to

supply a description of people's thoughts, feelings and perceptions. It does not set out to prove causal relationships nor test hypotheses as experimental research does. Examples of case studies include:

a description of how patients with multiple sclerosis cope with their disability;

an account of what it is like to train as a nurse on a three-year course.

Other designs are sometimes used in nursing research, including:

historical research;

philosophical research.

1 MAKING DECISIONS ABOUT METHODS

By the end of this section you will have discovered:

- exactly what you want to find out;
- what other people have discovered in this field and the methods they used to collect data.

Aim of the exercise To help you to state clearly what it is you want to find out in your research as a prerequisite of selecting the most appropriate method.

Planning stage You can do this exercise on your own or in the company of a small group of colleagues, friends or students. Allow yourself plenty of time to complete the exercise and make notes of what you do. If you work with friends or colleagues, decide whether you will all carry out similar tasks or whether you will divide up the work between you.

Equipment/resources required Notebook, pen and access to a nursing library.

EXERCISE 5.1

What to do Write *in one sentence* what your research is going to be about. Having clarified your ideas, go to the library and find three studies that have already explored aspects of the field of study that interests you. From those studies answer these questions:

- how did the researchers state the problem that they were researching?
- in what ways were the problems in those projects similar to your own?
- what methods of data collection did they use?
- in what ways will your research clarify the field or add to the body of knowledge?
- why are you choosing *this* problem?

Evaluation Discuss your research statement and the answers to the above questions with colleagues and with a tutor. Has the exercise made you modify your original research statement in any way or has it confirmed your need to pursue that line of research?

As another level of evaluation, it is useful, before you finish the activity, to note down:

(a) what you learned from doing the activity;
(b) how you will use what you learned;
(c) how what you have learned relates to what you have read;
(d) what you need to learn next.

2 IDENTIFYING THE RANGE OF AVAILABLE METHODS

By the end of this section you will have discovered:

● the range of research methods available to you.

Aim of the exercise To allow you to consider the range of possible data collection methods that will help you to answer your research question.

Planning stage You can do this exercise on your own or in the company of a small group of colleagues, friends or students. Allow yourself plenty of time to complete the exercise and make notes of what you do, as you go. If you work with friends or colleagues, decide whether you will all carry out similar tasks or whether you will divide up the work between you.

Equipment/resources required Notebook, pen and access to a nursing library.

EXERCISE 5.2

What to do Look through the following list of research methods and decide if each one is suitable, possibly suitable, or not suited to your project. If you do not have enough information to make a decision for any particular item then say so. The research methods you should consider for suitability include:

● questionnaire
● interview
● observation
● critical incident technique
● multiple sort/technique
● Delphi technique
● Q sort
● use of existing scales
● physiological measures
● projective techniques
● experiential research methods
● action research
● repertory grid technique
● use of existing records

Evaluation On what basis did you make your decisions? Do you have enough information to choose your method, at this stage, or do you need to do further studying? What does this exercise tell you about some of the problems of collecting data? What could you do to analyse this data?

As another level of evaluation, it is useful, before you finish the activity, to note down:

(a) what you learned from doing the activity;
(b) how you will use what you learned;
(c) how what you have learned relates to what you have read;
(d) what you need to learn next.

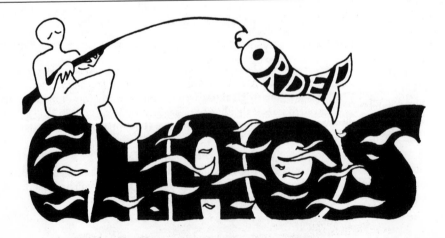

3 CHOOSING YOUR DATA COLLECTION METHOD

By the end of this section you will have discovered:

● how to choose a data collection method for your project.

EXERCISE 5.3

Aim of the exercise To enable you to make a choice about the method you will use to collect your research data.

Planning stage You can do this exercise on your own or in the company of a small group of colleagues, friends or students. Allow yourself plenty of time to complete the exercise and make notes of what you do. If you work with friends or colleagues, decide whether you will all carry out similar tasks or whether you will divide up the work between you.

Equipment/resources required Notebook, pen and access to a nursing library.

What to do Note the methods that you have selected from the last exercise as being suitable for your project. Now ask yourself the following questions about each method in order to be more clear about the choice you are going to make:

● do I know enough about the method?
  If not, go to the library, read more about the method and discuss it with your tutor.
● can I justify using this method rather than another?
  If not, is lack of knowledge about other methods the problem? Read about other methods.
● have I got the skills to carry out the method?
  If not, find out more about the skills from the library or from a tutor.
● is special equipment required to use this method?
  If so, do you have access to it? Can you get access?
● does the method take considerable time to use?
  If so, have you got the time within your time schedule?
● does the method require a large sample?
  If so, have you got access to the number required?
● do I know someone who has used this method and can give me support?
  If not, can you find someone?

Evaluation There are a number of questions that must be asked before you proceed with your project. Go to a tutor and ask to be questioned on your chosen method. Get a colleague to ask you awkward questions about the method. The final and most important question must be:
● is this method the most appropriate one for answering the research question?
  As another level of evaluation, it is useful, before you finish the activity, to note down:
(a) what you learned from doing the activity;
(b) how you will use what you learned;
(c) how what you have learned relates to what you have read;
(d) what you need to learn next.

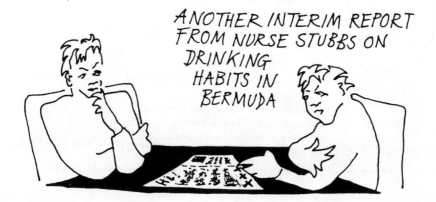

ANOTHER INTERIM REPORT FROM NURSE STUBBS ON DRINKING HABITS IN BERMUDA

4 CHOOSING YOUR METHOD OF DATA ANALYSIS

By the end of this section you will have discovered:

● the appropriate method for your research project.

It is vital that you consider how you will analyse your data as you collect it. This decision must be made alongside the decision about which data collection method you are going to use and not *after* that decision.

EXERCISE 5.4

Aim of the exercise To help you to select the most appropriate method of analysing your data.

Planning stage You can do this exercise on your own or in the company of a small group of colleagues, friends or students. Allow yourself plenty of time to complete the exercise and make notes of what you do. If you work with friends or colleagues, decide whether you will all carry out similar tasks or whether you will divide up the work between you.

Equipment/resources required Notebook, pen and access to a nursing library.

What to do Consider the following questions:

● are you going to have data which is easily converted into numbers?
● are you going to have data in the form of text?
● will your project lead to numbers and text?

If your project will lead you to numbers, consider the following questions:

● are you clear about how you will collect and store your data?
● do you have the necessary skills to perform the mathematics required in processing the data?
● if statistical tests are required, do you know which ones they are and can you use them?
● do you know how to *interpret* statistical data?
● do you know the limitations of using figures as data?
● how will you present your figures when you write your report?

Now read: Part Two; Selecting Methods of Data Collection; in Bell, J. (1987). *Doing Your Research Project: A Guide for First-Time Researchers in Education and Social Science*; Open University, Milton Keynes.
  If your project will lead you to text, consider the following questions:

● are you clear about how you will collect and store your data?
● do you have the necessary skills to analyse and categorise the data?
● where can you obtain further advice on handling textual data?
● what psychological, sociological or political theories will guide your analysis?
● do you know how to interpret any findings?
● do you know the limitations of using raw text as data?
● how will you present your data when you write your report?

Now read: Turner, B. A. (1981). Some Practical Aspects of Qualitative Data Analysis: One Way of Organising Some of the Cognitive Processes Associated With the Generation of Grounded Theory; *Quality and Quantity*, 15, 225–247.

Evaluation Discuss your work with your colleagues and with your tutor.
  As another level of evaluation, it is useful, before you finish the activity, to note down:
(a) what you learned from doing the activity;
(b) how you will use what you learned;
(c) how what you have learned relates to what you have read;
(d) what you need to learn next.

INFORMATION BOX

Pilot studies

Now that you have considered a variety of methods of collecting data, you will want to try out some methods. This will lead to a pilot study.

A pilot study is a small-scale version of the research project which allows you to test out your data collection method. The pilot study should point up deficiencies in your planning and will allow you to smooth them out. The pilot study may also show you that the method chosen is not suitable for the project. In this case you may need to consider other methods. You will have to conduct another pilot study and the details of all pilot studies should be written into your final research report.

Time spent on pilot studies can pay great dividends later on. Some of the questions that a pilot study will allow you to consider are:

can the respondents understand what is being asked of them?

does the data collection method collect the sort of data required?

is there *time* to use this method?

are there ethical problems associated with this method?

what revisions are required to modify the plan?

CONCLUSION

You should now feel confident about how you want to conduct your research project. In the following chapters we will consider the issues of method and analysis.

LEARNING CHECK

If you are a working on your own

● Read through the notes you made while completing the exercises in this chapter and consider the following questions:
  – What new knowledge have I gained?
  – What new skills have I developed?
  – How has my thinking about research changed?
  – What do I need to do now?
● Check that you have made reference cards for any new references that you have found whilst working on the exercises in this chapter.

If you are working in a small group

● Pair off and nominate one of you as A and one of you as B. For five minutes, A talks to B about what has been learned and B listens. This should not be a conversation: B's only role is to listen. After five minutes, roles are reversed and B talks to A about what has been learned and A listens. After the second five minutes, re-form into a group and discuss the experience.

If you are a tutor and/or facilitator

● Use the above 'pairs' exercise with the group you are working with.
● Hold two 'rounds' in which each person in turn says what was liked *least* about doing the activities and what was liked *most* about doing the activities.

6 · METHODS OF COLLECTING DATA

WHAT YOU NEED TO READ

Bryman, A. (1988). *Quantity and Quality in Social Research*, Unwin Hyman, London.

Darling, V. H. and Rogers, J. (1986). *Research for Practising Nurses*, Macmillan, Basingstoke.

Long, A. F. (1984). *Research into Health and Illness: Issues in Design, Analysis and Practice*, Gower, Aldershot.

Watson, J. (1985). *Nursing: Human Science and Human Care: A Theory of Nursing*, Appleton-Century-Crofts, Norwalk, Connecticut.

AIMS OF THIS CHAPTER

- To explore four methods of data collection;
- To identify the strengths and weaknesses of each method;
- To enable you to consider the usefulness of these methods for your research project.

INTRODUCTION

In this chapter we look at specific data collection methods. You will have already decided what methods you are likely to use but it may be useful to read through this chapter and do the exercises. This will familiarise you with other systems and you may find that you want to change your data collection method. This chapter deals with those methods that are well established. Traditional ways of finding out information tend to have been by means of:

- structured interviews;
- questionnaires;
- experiments;
- observation.

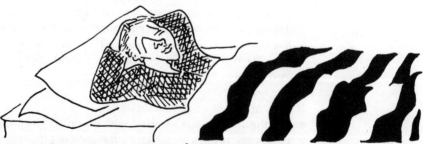

IN 1920 OTTO LOEWI DISCOVERED THE CHEMICAL TRANSMISSION OF NERVE IMPULSES IN A DREAM

INFORMATION BOX

Validity and reliability

Methods used for data collection must be valid and reliable. Validity refers to whether or not a method measures what it sets out to measure. Reliability refers to the issue of whether or not a method works consistently.

There are different questions about validity and reliability to be addressed in using quantitative and qualitative approaches to research. Therefore, the reader is recommended to read the following references on the issues of validity and reliability.

- Le Compte, M. D. and Goetz, J. P. (1982). Problems of Reliability and Validity in Ethnographic Research; *Review of Educational Research*, 52, **1**, 31–60.
- Sapsford, R. J. and Evans, J. (1984). Evaluating a Research Report; in J. Bell, T. Bush, A. Fox, J. Goodey and S. Golding (eds) (1984). *Conducting Small-Scale Investigations in Educational Management*; Harper and Row, London.
- Waltz, C. F., Strickland, O. L. and Lenz, E. R. (1984). *Measurement in Nursing Research*; F. A. Davis, Philadelphia.
- Wertz, F. J. (1986). The Question of the Reliability of Psychological Research; *Journal of Phenomenological Psychology*, 17, **2**, 181–205.

INFORMATION BOX

Sampling methods

The purpose of research is to explore various themes and trends throughout a certain population of people. It is usually impractical to attempt to collect data from every member of that population. Therefore it is necessary to choose a *sample* from that population. A sample is a group of people from a larger population. A sample may also be a collection of records or a number of observations, for example. Ideally you should select a sample of people that is representative of the larger group. There are various ways of selecting a sample. These include:

simple random sampling
stratified random sampling
cluster sampling
opportunistic sampling
quota sampling
convenience sampling
strategic informant sampling
purposive sampling
snowball sampling.

The sample that you need for your study will be determined to a large degree by what you are researching, what methods you are using and the time you have available. You need to discuss the question of sampling with your tutor or lecturer.

You may find the following references useful when considering how to select a sample:
- Field, P. A. and Morse, J. M. (1985). *Nursing Research: The Application of Qualitative Approaches*; Croom Helm, London.
- Reid, N. G. and Boore, J. R. P. (1987). *Research Methods and Statistics in Health Care*; Arnold, London.
- Smith, H. W. (1981). *Strategies of Social Research: The Methodological Imagination*; 2nd Edition, Prentice Hall, Englewood Cliffs, New Jersey.

1 STRUCTURED INTERVIEWS

You will need to know the following:

- what a structured interview is;
- the difference between a structured interview and an unstructured interview;
- how to analyse a structured interview;
- the limitations of using a structured interview.

EXERCISE 6.1

Aim of the exercise To explore the use of the unstructured interview.

Planning stage This activity needs to be carried out with at least one other person: a colleague or a friend. Allow yourself plenty of time to complete the exercise and make notes of what you do, as you go.

Equipment/resources required Notebook, pen, access to a nursing library, tape recorder.

What to do Without any preparation ask a friend to tell you about his/her work. Encourage the flow of conversation by asking any questions that come to mind and which have a bearing on the topic. Make notes about your colleague's responses or make a tape recording of the interview. If you can, repeat the process with one other friend.

Evaluation When you have completed each interview, ask yourself the following questions about the data you collected:

- do you have a detailed account of your colleague's work?
- did the conversation flow in an orderly manner and have a beginning, a middle and an end?
- how much did I talk during the interview?
- to what degree did I influence the answers?
- could I have collected the data more effectively?

As another level of evaluation, it is useful, before you finish the activity, to note down:
(a) what you learned from doing the activity;
(b) how you will use what you learned;
(c) how what you have learned relates to what you have read;
(d) what you need to learn next.

EXERCISE 6.2

Aim of the exercise To devise a short structured interview schedule and to use this as a basis for carrying out an interview.

Planning stage This activity needs to be carried out with at least one other person: a colleague or a friend. Allow yourself plenty of time to complete the exercise and make notes of what you do, as you go.

Equipment/resources required Notebook, pen and access to a nursing library.

What to do Write out ten questions that you would like to ask a colleague about his/her job. Ask your colleague the questions and note down the answers. If possible, repeat the process with one or more colleagues.

Evaluation Look at the replies and ask yourself the following questions:

- did my questions get answers I anticipated?
- how will I analyse the answers I was offered?
- how could I improve my interview schedule?

Discuss your questions and the answers with someone who has used a structured/*resources* interview approach. Produce a list of the pros and cons of the unstructured and structured approaches to interviewing.

As another level of evaluation, it is useful, before you finish the activity, to note down:
(a) what you learned from doing the activity;
(b) how you will use what you learned;
(c) how what you have learned relates to what you have read;
(d) what you need to learn next.

INFORMATION BOX

Open and closed questions

Closed questions are those that lead to a restricted range of answers such as 'yes' or 'no'. Examples of closed questions are:

do you smoke?

how satisfied are you with your present state of health? Choose from very satisfied, satisfied, dissatisfied.

Open questions are those that lead to answers which cannot be anticipated and are usually lengthy. Open questions usually begin with what, why, where or how. Examples of open questions are:

what are your views on smoking?

why are you dissatisfied with your health?

Closed and open questions may be used in research interviews. Structured interviews that use closed questions may be analysed quantitatively. Unstructured interviews that use open questions may be analysed qualitatively. In between these two extremes are semi-structured interviews that may combine open and closed questions about the same topic.

2 QUESTIONNAIRES

Questionnaires differ from structured interviews by the degree of personal involvement on the part of the researcher at the point of data collection.

You will need to know the following:

● what a questionnaire is;
● what types of questionnaire exist;
● what the advantages and disadvantages of questionnaires are.

Aim of the exercise To become familiar with various types of questionnaires.

Planning stage The exercise can be carried out alone or with a group of colleagues. Allow yourself plenty of time to complete the exercise and make notes of what you do. If you work with friends or colleagues, decide whether you will all carry out similar tasks or whether you will divide up the work between you.

Equipment/resources required Notebook, pen and access to a nursing library.

EXERCISE 6.3

What to do Write a short questionnaire which will provide answers to the following:

● is nursing stressful?
● are some nurses more assertive than others?
● do nurses use a nursing model in their practice?

When you have written your questions, go to the library and find the following books:

– Converse, J. M. and Presser, S. (1986). *Survey Questions: Handcrafting the Standardised Questionnaire*; Sage, Beverly Hills.
– Oppenheim, A. N. (1966). *Questionnaire Design and Attitude Measurement*; Heinemann, London.
– Sudman, S. and Bradburn, N. M. (1987). *Asking Questions: A Practical Guide to Questionnaire Design*; Jossey Bass, San Francisco.

Read through the sections on questionnaires and answer the following:

● what is a questionnaire?
● what is the purpose of a questionnaire?
● what distinguishes a questionnaire from an interview?
● how can you analyse the data from questionnaires?
● what principles go into the production of questionnaires?

Now read through your own questions and see if they need to be modified.

continued

Evaluation Try out your modified questionnaire on a friend. Ask if there are any objections to the construction of your questionnaire. Also, show the questionnaire to a tutor and ask his/her opinion of your work.

If you worked in a group, share your experiences and see if problems were common.

As another level of evaluation, it is useful, before you finish the activity, to note down:

(a) what you learned from doing the activity;
(b) how you will use what you learned;
(c) how what you have learned relates to what you have read;
(d) what you need to learn next.

INFORMATION BOX

Advantages and disadvantages of questionnaires

Advantages	*Disadvantages*
A straightforward way of collecting data quickly and efficiently;	No personal contact with respondents;
Cheap to use;	Can be difficult to construct;
Allow the researcher to collect information anonymously;	Involve 'forced choice' of response;
Easy to analyse;	Cannot probe in-depth issues.
Can handle large batches of data.	

---

3 EXPERIMENTS

Experiments are systematic attempts to test an hypothesis. Experimental research attempts to identify causal relationships between variables and tries to establish 'laws'. Few nurses just starting research will be planning experimental studies. However, it is useful to be able to understand experimental studies.

You will need to know the following:

- what forms an hypothesis;
- some of the terms associated with experimental research;
- how to become critical of experimental research reports.

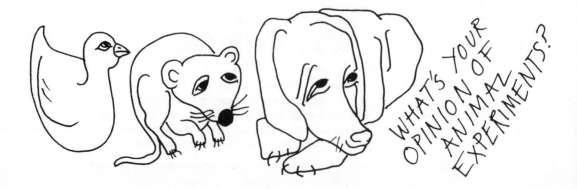

WHAT'S YOUR OPINION OF ANIMAL EXPERIMENTS?

EXERCISE 6.4

Aim of the exercise To explore the notions of hypothesis and null hypothesis.

Planning stage This activity can be carried out alone, or with a group of colleagues. Allow yourself plenty of time to complete the exercise and make notes of what you do. If you work with friends or colleagues, decide whether you will all carry out similar tasks or whether you will divide up the work between you.

Equipment/resources required Notebook, pen, access to a nursing library, tape recorder.

What to do Go to the library and find the books listed below. Read through the sections on hypotheses which are found on the page numbers referenced.
– Dixon, B. R., Bouma, G. D. and Atkinson, G. B. J. (1987). *A Handbook of Social Science Research: A Comprehensive and Practical Guide for Students*; Oxford University Press, Oxford, p. 53–58.
– Leedy, P. D. (1985). *Practical Research: Planning and Design*; 3rd Edition, Macmillan, New York, p. 5–6 and 64–65.

Evaluation Ask yourself the following questions:

● what is an hypothesis?
● what is a null hypothesis?
● how do you use an hypothesis?
● what is the difference between an hypothesis and an assumption?
● what does the term 'variable' mean?

Now talk to your tutor about the concept of hypotheses.
   As another level of evaluation, it is useful, before you finish the activity, to note down:
(a) what you learned from doing the activity;
(b) how you will use what you learned;
(c) how what you have learned relates to what you have read;
(d) what you need to learn next.

EXERCISE 6.5

Aim of the exercise To explore some of the terms commonly used in experimental research.

Planning stage This activity can be carried out alone, or with a group of colleagues. Allow yourself plenty of time to complete the exercise and make notes of what you do. If you work with friends or colleagues, decide whether you will all carry out similar tasks or whether you will divide up the work between you.

Equipment/resources required Notebook, pen, access to a nursing library.

What to do Read books on research and write some definitions for the terms listed below. You will find a list of suitable books in the back of this one.

● control group
● experimental group
● statistical significance
● sampling
● confounding variables

Now read the following two research reports and note how these terms are used.
– Hayward, J. (1975). *Information: A Prescription Against Pain*; Royal College of Nursing, London.
– Luker, K. A. (1982). *Evaluating Health Visiting Practice*; Royal College of Nursing, London.

Evaluation Discuss the above terms with friends and with a tutor to make sure you understand the words.
   As another level of evaluation, it is useful, before you finish the activity, to note down:
(a) what you learned from doing the activity;
(b) how you will use what you learned;
(c) how what you have learned relates to what you have read;
(d) what you need to learn next.

4 OBSERVATION

By the end of this section you will have discovered:

● what sort of information is being sought through observation;
● some of the problems associated with observation;
● what types of observational methods can be used.

EXERCISE 6.6

Aim of the exercise To explore problems and practical issues associated with observation.

Planning stage You can do this exercise on your own or in the company of a small group of colleagues, friends or students. Allow yourself plenty of time to complete the exercise and make notes of what you do. If you work with friends or colleagues, decide whether you will all carry out similar tasks or whether you will divide up the work between you.

Equipment/resources required Notebook, pen and access to a nursing library.

What to do Go to somewhere crowded or busy such as a bus station, an out-patients' department or a staff cafeteria. Sit and observe people for about ten minutes and make notes. Now answer the following questions:

● what sort of things did you see?
● how did you decide what to observe and what to ignore?
● how did you make notes on what you observed?
● did you try to interpret what people were doing and why?

By answering these questions you are beginning to appreciate the difficulties faced by researchers when trying to decide how to collect data by observation.

Now repeat your short study but before you begin observing identify what you want to observe. You might be interested in how many people get on a particular bus when it stops at a bus station or you might want to observe how many people choose salad as a meal in the staff cafeteria, for example.

To help in your observation, draw up a simple checklist on which you can record what you see. Now go back to the crowded place for a further ten minutes and use your checklist to record your second observation.

Now ask yourself the following questions:

● was the second period of observation easier or more difficult than the first?
● did your checklist help or hinder you?
● did your checklist work?

Now read the following to help you understand how observational methods may be used to collect research data.

– Henerson, M. E., Morris, L. L. and Fitz-Gibbon, C. T. (1987). *How to Measure Attitudes*; Sage, Beverly Hills, California, chapter 9.
– Lofland, J. and Lofland, L. (1984). *Analysing Social Settings*; 2nd Edition, Wadsworth, Newark, New Jersey.
– Taylor, S. J. and Bogdan, R. (1984). *Introduction to Qualitative Research Methods: The Search for Meanings*; 2nd Edition, Wiley, New York.

Evaluation If you are working in a small group, discuss your findings with your colleagues.

As another level of evaluation, it is useful, before you finish the activity, to note down:

(a) what you learned from doing the activity;
(b) how you will use what you learned;
(c) how what you have learned relates to what you have read;
(d) what you need to learn next.

INFORMATION BOX

Aspects of observation in research

There are two types of observation—participant and non-participant. In non-participant observation the researcher enters a setting as an observer and records examples of behaviour or action. No attempt is made to influence the situation. Of course, the presence of the researcher *may* change what is happening. In participant observation the researcher enters a situation and works alongside the people involved. You may want to consider the pros and cons of these two approaches and think about possible ethical problems. In any event observation must be specific, recorded quickly and accurately as well as being informative.

CONCLUSION

In this chapter we have considered four main types of data collection methods. If you can become familiar with the main skills involved in each of these methods you will be able to examine the research literature more critically. You may find, however, that the methods explored in this chapter are not suited to your own research project, in which case those of the next chapter may offer more scope.

LEARNING CHECK

If you are a working on your own
- Read through the notes you made while completing the exercises in this chapter and consider the following questions:
  - What new knowledge have I gained?
  - What new skills have I developed?
  - How has my thinking about research changed?
  - What do I need to do now?
- Check that you have made reference cards for any new references that you have found whilst working on the exercises in this chapter.

If you are working in a small group
- Pair off and nominate one of you as A and one of you as B. For five minutes, A talks to B about what has been learned and B listens. This should not be a conversation: B's only role is to listen. After five minutes, roles are reversed and B talks to A about what has been learned and A listens. After the second five minutes, re-form into a group and discuss the experience.

If you are a tutor and/or facilitator
- Use the above 'pairs' exercise with the group you are working with.
- Hold two 'rounds' in which each person in turn says what was liked *least* about doing the activities and what was liked *most* about doing the activities.

7 ◆ OTHER METHODS OF COLLECTING DATA

WHAT YOU NEED TO READ

Field, P. A. and Morse, J. M. (1985). *Nursing Research: The Application of Qualitative Approaches*, Croom Helm, London.

Sweener, M. A. and Oliveri, P. (1981). *An Introduction to Nursing Research: Research, Measurement and Computers in Nursing*, J. B. Lipincott, Philadelphia.

Van Maanen, J. (1983). *Qualitative Methodology*, Sage, Beverly Hills, California.

Verhonick, P. and Seaman, C. (1978). *Research Methods for Undergraduate Students in Nursing*, Appleton-Century-Crofts, New York.

AIMS OF THIS CHAPTER

- To look at a variety of other research data collection methods;
- To consider the usefulness of these methods for your project;
- To identify key references for further reading.

INTRODUCTION

In the last chapter we considered four common methods of collecting data. In this chapter we consider some other methods that you may want to use. There is no right or wrong way of collecting data. Different projects, different research questions and different levels of experience will influence the decision to choose one method rather than another. Choosing the right method is the key to success. In this chapter we consider the following additional methods of research:

- use of existing records;
- repertory grid technique;
- critical incident technique;
- multiple sort;
- use of existing scales, inventories, tests and assessment tools;
- semantic differential.

This is not an exhaustive list of data collection techniques and you are advised to look for other methods not covered in this book.

I USE OF EXISTING RECORDS

By the end of this section you will have discovered:

- what sort of records can be used in a research project;
- how to gain access to records;
- how to use records in research.

Aim of the exercise To explore the use of data collected from existing records.

Planning stage You can do this exercise on your own or in the company of a small group of colleagues, friends or students. Allow yourself plenty of time to complete the exercise and make notes of what you do. If you work with friends or colleagues, decide whether you will all carry out similar tasks or whether you will divide up the work between you.

Equipment/resources required Notebook, pen and access to a nursing library.

EXERCISE 7.1

What to do Ask a senior nurse if you may have access to one of the sets of records listed below. Explain why you want to look at them and say that you will destroy your written work after you have completed the exercise.

- off duty sheets for the past month;
- the accident book on your ward;
- ward report sheets for the past month.

Make a note of the type of information that is contained in the records you are investigating. Devise a simple method of collecting some of the information on to one sheet of paper. Look through the data you have collected and see if any particular patterns are apparent. Gradually, you will produce a mental picture of the trends and patterns contained within the data. This approach to working with records can lead you to ask other questions about the topic in which you are interested and can point your research in other directions.

Evaluation Discuss your findings in your small group and see to what degree there is agreement about trends and patterns emerging out of the data.

As another level of evaluation, it is useful, before you finish the activity, to note down:
(a) what you learned from doing the activity;
(b) how you will use what you learned;
(c) how what you have learned relates to what you have read;
(d) what you need to learn next.

2 REPERTORY GRID TECHNIQUE

By the end of this section you will have discovered:

- how to consider using Kelly's repertory grid technique.

INFORMATION BOX

Personal construct theory and repertory grids

The repertory grid technique is based on the personal construct theory. In its simplest form this seeks to identify the characteristics that an individual looks for in other people and in his/her immediate environment. These characteristics are called 'constructs' and the originator of the theory, George Kelly, argued that they are usually two-sided. A person who sees some individuals as 'caring' will also see others as 'uncaring'. Kelly also argued that constructs vary from person to person.

Kelly used the word 'element' to describe people, events and items viewed by individuals. It is possible to consider three elements and to consider the ways two of those elements differ from the third. For example, you may consider a doctor and nurse to be professionals while a ward visitor is not a professional. Alternatively, you may consider that the nurse and the visitor are approachable but the doctor is distant. In these examples the visitor, doctor and nurse are elements and the descriptions professional and distant – not professional and approachable – are both bipolar constructs.

This approach to identifying ways individuals view others and the world around them can be exploited for the purposes of research. The approach may be used to find out how a group of nurses perceives working in an accident and emergency unit, for

continued

example, or how they feel about their colleagues, their work, their training and so on. Much has been written about the personal construct approach and the use of the repertory grid technique in research. The following contain useful information:

– Bannister, D. and Fransella, F. (1986). *Inquiring Man*; 3rd Edition, Croom Helm, London.
– Beail, N. (1985). An Introduction to Repertory Grid Technique; in Beail N. (ed) (1985). *Repertory Grid Technique and Personal Constructs*; Croom Helm, London, p. 1–24.
– Pollock, L. C. (1986). An Introduction to the Use of Repertory Grid Technique as a Research Method and Clinical Tool for Psychiatric Nurses; *Journal of Advanced Nursing*, 11, 439–445.
– Stewart, V. and Stewart, A. (1981). *Business Applications of Repertory Grid*; McGraw Hill, London.

EXERCISE 7.2

Aim of the exercise To explore some basic principles of the repertory grid technique.

Planning stage You can do this exercise on your own or in the company of a small group of colleagues, friends or students. Allow yourself plenty of time to complete the exercise and make notes of what you do. If you work with friends or colleagues, decide whether you will all carry out similar tasks or whether you will divide up the work between you.

Equipment/resources required Notebook, pen and access to a nursing library.

What to do Consider the following list of types of people and write down a name for each one. The list you produce is a selection of 'elements' for you to consider.

● a good friend
● your mother
● your father
● a favourite teacher
● someone you don't like
● yourself

Now think about the elements you have listed. Consider them in groups of three and identify ways in which two of the people are similar and different from the third. Write down the similarities and the differences for each group of three. This will produce a list of bipolar constructs and will offer you some ideas about how you view others.

Now consider the range of personal constructs you have produced. Are you surprised by the constructs or are they representative of the sorts of qualities you thought you attributed to other people?

Evaluation If you are working in a small group, discuss your findings with your colleagues. Also, consider ways that you may use this approach in a research project.

As another level of evaluation, it is useful, before you finish the activity, to note down:
(a) what you learned from doing the activity;
(b) how you will use what you learned;
(c) how what you have learned relates to what you have read;
(d) what you need to learn next.

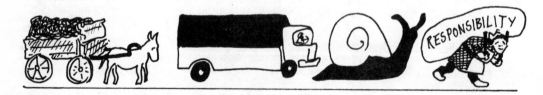

3 CRITICAL INCIDENT TECHNIQUE

By the end of this section you will have discovered:

● how the critical incident technique is used in research.

INFORMATION BOX

Critical incident technique

The critical incident technique offers the opportunity to study how people describe their reactions in certain situations. For example, it may be useful to find out how nursing assistants feel about their reactions to a patient having a cardiac arrest. The technique may also be used to discover how different groups of people say they reacted in particular situations. For example, it may be interesting to find out how doctors, senior nurses and nursing assistants feel about their actions when a patient has a cardiac arrest.

The critical incident technique is used to help people to reflect on past events and to note how they report their reactions. Different methods of data collection may be used to gather examples of incidents for review and for identifying people's perceptions of those incidents. For example, the researcher may use interviews, questionnaires, records or self-report measures.

The analysis of the data obtained involves the classification of responses to incidents. For example, ward sisters may be asked to think of a time when they were functioning particularly well in their role as teacher. The words and phrases that they use to describe their performance are then filtered into a variety of categories such as 'effective communication', 'skilled behaviour', 'enjoyment' and so on. These categories can then be used to present the data in a written format and they may allow the researcher to offer answers to the research question.

For further details of how to use the critical incident technique, see:
- Cormack, D. F. S. (1983). *Psychiatric Nursing Described*; Churchill Livingstone, Edinburgh.
- Cormack, D. F. S. (1984). Flanagan's Critical Incident Technique; in Cormack, D. F. S. (ed) (1984). *The Research Process in Nursing*; Blackwell, Oxford, p. 118–125.
- Flanagan, J. C. (1954). The Critical Incident Technique; *Psychological Bulletin*, 51, 4, 327–358.

Aim of the exercise To explore one aspect of the critical incident technique.

Planning stage You can do this exercise on your own or in the company of a small group of colleagues, friends or students. Allow yourself plenty of time to complete the exercise. If you work with friends or colleagues, decide whether you will all carry out similar tasks or divide up the work between you.

Equipment/resources required Notebook, pen and access to a nursing library.

continued

EXERCISE 7.3

What to do Consider one of the following incidents from your past:

● observing a patient having an epileptic fit;
● the fire alarm sounding when you were at work;
● giving a patient an injection;
● being present at a road traffic accident.

Now write down what happened and write down what you did. Answer the following questions:

● do you consider that your action was appropriate? If not, why not?
● how did you feel about what happened?
● in what ways could your performance have been improved?
● what did you learn from the incident?
● what would you do differently next time?

Now look through your replies and see if any trends occur and if they can be placed under broad headings.

Evaluation If you are working in a small group, share experiences and reactions. Do your reactions fall into certain categories and can you agree, as a group, on the categories generated by this activity?

As another level of evaluation, it is useful, before you finish the activity, to note down:

(a) what you learned from doing the activity;
(b) how you will use what you learned;
(c) how what you have learned relates to what you have read;
(d) what you need to learn next.

4 MULTIPLE SORT

By the end of this section you will have discovered:

● how to consider using the multiple sort technique in a research project.

EXERCISE 7.4

Aim of the exercise To explore the use of the multiple sort technique.

Planning stage This exercise involves two people—you as the researcher and a colleague as the informant. Allow yourself plenty of time to complete the exercise and make notes of what you do.

Equipment/resources required Small pieces of paper or card, notebook, pen and access to a nursing library.

What to do Write the following phrases on separate cards:

psychiatric nursing
geriatric nursing
paediatric nursing
orthopaedic nursing
ophthalmic nursing
oncology nursing
mental handicap nursing
medical nursing
surgical nursing

cardiac nursing
midwifery
health visiting
district nursing
community psychiatric nursing
school nursing
occupational health nursing
industrial nursing

Now ask your colleague to look through the cards and sort them into piles. Your colleague is free to determine how the cards are divided. Then ask your colleague to label the piles. Make a note of the labels and the cards in each pile. Now sort the cards yourself. See whether or not you produce a different set of piles or a different number of piles.

In doing this exercise you have been using the multiple sort technique, which allows you to explore another person's viewpoint and style of differentiating between items. For further information, see:

– Canter, D., Brown, J. and Groat, L. (1985). A Multiple Sorting Procedure for Studying Conceptual Systems; in Brenner, M., Brown, J. and Canter, D. (eds) (1985). *The Research Interview: Uses and Approaches*; Academic Press, London, p. 79–114.
– Groat, L. (1982). Meaning in Post-Modern Architecture: An Examination Using the Multiple Sorting Task; *Journal of Environmental Psychology*, 2, 3, 3–22.

Evaluation Discuss the groups of cards and their labels with your colleague and discuss ways that the method could be used in a research project.

As another level of evaluation, it is useful, before you finish the activity, to note down:

(a) what you learned from doing the activity;
(b) how you will use what you learned;
(c) how what you have learned relates to what you have read;
(d) what you need to learn next.

5 USE OF EXISTING SCALES, INVENTORIES, TESTS AND ASSESSMENT TOOLS

By the end of this section you will have discovered:

● how to find existing scales, inventories, tests and assessment tools;
● whether or not such scales, inventories, tests or assessment tools would be useful in your research project.

Aim of the exercise To explore the use of existing scales, inventories and assessment tools.

Planning stage You can do this exercise on your own or in the company of a small group of colleagues, friends or students. Allow yourself plenty of time to complete the exercise and make notes of what you do. If you work with friends or colleagues, decide whether you will all carry out similar tasks or whether you will divide up the work between you.

Equipment/resources required Notebook, pen and access to a nursing library.

EXERCISE 7.5

What to do Go to the library and locate one or more of the following references, which provide established sources of scales, inventories, tests or assessment tools:
– Anastasi, A. (1988). *Psychological Testing*; 6th Edition, Macmillan, New York.
– Robinson, J. P. and Shaver, P. R. (1973). *Measures of Social Psychological Attitudes*; Institute for Social Research, University of Michigan, Ann Arbor, Michigan.
– Ward, M. J. and Felter, M. E. (1979). *Instruments for Use in Nursing Education Research*; Western Interstate Commission for Higher Education, Boulder, Colorado.

If you have difficulty in obtaining these publications choose alternatives from the list of scales, inventories, tests and assessment tools in the Compendium of useful information at the back of this book.

Scan through two of the instruments that you have found and answer the following questions:

● how was the instrument developed?
● how was it tested?
● does the instrument relate specifically to nursing? If not, could it be used in a nursing context?
● does the instrument relate to a particular culture or does it claim to be applicable across a wide range of cultures?
● is it suitable for your particular needs?
● if you were to use it, would you need permission?
● could you analyse the data obtained?

Evaluation Discuss your findings with a group of colleagues. If you find that you do want to use a particular instrument, discuss its use with a tutor first. You may be surprised at how many instruments have already been defined. Also, you may be able to adapt an existing instrument to suit your particular needs. If a suitable instrument does exist you may be advised to use it, rather than spend considerable time devising your own.

As another level of evaluation, it is useful, before you finish the activity, to note down:
(a) what you learned from doing the activity;
(b) how you will use what you learned;
(c) how what you have learned relates to what you have read;
(d) what you need to learn next.

6 SEMANTIC DIFFERENTIAL

By the end of this section you will have discovered:

● what forms the semantic differential technique;
● whether or not you could use it in your research project.

INFORMATION BOX

Semantic differential technique

Semantic differential explores the ways that people use words to describe situations. It is a highly structured means of exploring perceptions of situations, people or things. If we accept that each of us views a situation slightly differently and that we use a variety of words to describe that situation then it may be useful to find out more about different sets of words and meanings.

The semantic differential approach allows a researcher to explore the similarities and the differences between perceptions of situation, people and things. It is an underlying assumption of the technique, that certain words have similar meanings for different individuals.

The technique offers subjects a series of bipolar dimensions along which they rate themselves, other people or activities. For example, a subject may be asked to consider his/her ability to care. This is done by placing a tick on a scale like the one below. Ratings along the scale can be compared.

caring |__|__|__|__|__|__|*uncaring*

For further information about the semantic differential approach, see the following:

– Choon, G. L. and Skevington, S. M. (1984). How do Women and Men in Nursing Perceive each Other? in Skevington, S. (ed) (1984). *Understanding Nurses*; Wiley, Chichester p. 101–111.
– Kerlinger, F. N. (1986). *Foundations of Behavioural Research*; 3rd Edition, CBS Publishing, Tokyo.
– Osgood, C. E., Suci, G. J. and Tannenbaum, P. H. (1957). *The Measurement of Meaning*; University of Illinois Press, Urbana, Illinois.

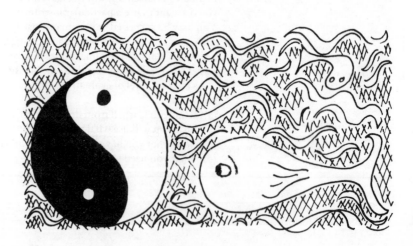

EXERCISE 7.6

Aim of the exercise To explore the use of the semantic differential approach.

Planning stage This exercise is initially to be carried out by you working alone, yet in the company of others. In the evaluation stage, it is important that you work with a small group of colleagues. Allow yourself plenty of time to complete the exercise and make notes of what you do.

Equipment/resources required Notebook, pen and access to a nursing library.

What to do Consider the following dimensions and rate your own perception on the scale provided, by placing ticks at the most appropriate points.

Your perceptions of a person with AIDS

A person with AIDS may be

Weak								Powerful
Conformist								Non-conformist
Dominant								Submissive
Aggressive								Peaceful
Kind								Unkind
Logical								Intuitive
Stupid								Intelligent
Clean								Unclean
Happy								Sad
Moral								Immoral

Now draw a line that links up all the pencil marks and create a profile of how you perceive AIDS patients. This will allow you to spot similarities and differences when you compare your ratings with those of your colleagues. The ticks on each dimension may also be given a numerical value, which would make analysis easier. Statistical analysis could be used to process the data and establish precise differences between individuals and groups of subjects.

Evaluation Discuss and compare your findings with those of your colleagues. How could you analyse data collected from a group of people? Is this a method that you could use in your own research project?

As another level of evaluation, it is useful, before you finish the activity, to note down:
(a) what you learned from doing the activity;
(b) how you will use what you learned;
(c) how what you have learned relates to what you have read;
(d) what you need to learn next.

OBSERVATION NOW YOU SEE ME JUDGEMENT
CRITICISM NOW YOU DON'T VALUE
DESCRIPTION PERCEPTION
FACT OPINION
DEFINITION SUPPOSITION

INFORMATION BOX

Other methods to consider

The *Delphi Method* is used to quantify the judgments of experts, to assess priorities, or to produce long-range forecasts. The Delphi Method is useful as a means of:

gathering current and historical data not accurately known or available;

examining the significance of historical events;

evaluating possible budget options;

exploring planning options;

planning curriculum developments;

looking at the pros and cons of policy options.

The Delphi Method involves asking a group of experts to offer information about a particular topic. Out of the material that is generated a questionnaire is developed which is sent out to that same panel of experts. This cyclical process is continued until the researcher feels confident that a comprehensive view of the field has been obtained. The aim is to produce an outcome that is acceptable to the panel of experts.

A useful source of further information about the Delphi Method is:

– Fielding, G. (1984). Professional Problems of Caring for the Cancer Patient; *International Review of Applied Psychology*, 33, 545–563.

The *case study* approach looks at individuals in a problematic situation over a short period of time. It is a word-picture of one part of a person's life. Examples of the case study would be a description of an individual's care and experience during treatment for cancer, or a description of a manager's experience of being displaced during a reorganisation.

Case studies offer a 'one off' approach to data collection. They offer a rich source of qualitative and descriptive data which can be analysed later. Many nurses are familiar with being asked to prepare a case study. For research, a case study would be of greater depth than most nurses usually write. Considerably more detail would be required in a research case study and the analysis of the data would be more stringent.

A useful book on this topic is:

– Bromley, D. B. (1986). *The Case Study Method in Psychology and Related Disciplines*; Wiley, Chichester.

Diaries and journals are descriptions of activities, experiences and feelings, written during a particular time-span. For example, a group of ward sisters may be asked to keep a diary of their work activities for a period of two months. The information gained in this way can be a rich source of descriptive data. This method is an example of self-reporting. A useful discussion of the pros and cons of this method is offered in:

– Henerson, M. E., Morris, L. L. and Fitz-Gibbon, C. T. (1987). *How to Measure Attitudes*; Sage, Beverly Hills, California.

CONCLUSION

There is a variety of alternative methods of data collection. They have not necessarily been used as frequently in nursing research as those described in the previous chapter but all are interesting and valuable. The overriding principle in selecting a method is that it should be the one that provides the data you need to answer your research question. It is wise to become familiar with a wide range of methods and to note how other researchers have chosen their methods. In this way you will gradually become more critical of the work of other investigators—a vital aspect of the research process.

LEARNING CHECK

If you are a working on your own
● Read through the notes you made while completing the exercises in this chapter and consider the following questions:
 – What new knowledge have I gained?
 – What new skills have I developed?
 – How has my thinking about research changed?
 – What do I need to do now?
● Check that you have made reference cards for any new references that you have found whilst working on the exercises in this chapter.

If you are working in a small group
● Pair off and nominate one of you as A and one of you as B. For five minutes, A talks to B about what has been learned and B listens. This should not be a conversation: B's only role is to listen. After five minutes, roles are reversed and B talks to A about what has been learned and A listens. After the second five minutes, re-form into a group and discuss the experience.

If you are a tutor and/or facilitator
● Use the above 'pairs' exercise with the group you are working with.
● Hold two 'rounds' in which each person in turn says what was liked *least* about doing the activities and what was liked *most* about doing the activities.

8 ◆ METHODS OF ANALYSING DATA

WHAT YOU NEED TO READ

Burgess, R. G. (1984). *In the Field: An Introduction to Field Research*, Allen and Unwin, London.

Goulding, S. (1987). Analysis and Presentation of Information; in Bell, J. (1987). *Doing Your Research Project: A Guide for First-Time Researchers in Education and Social Science*, Open University Press, Milton Keynes; p. 103–123.

Lofland, J. and Lofland, L. (1984). *Analysing Social Settings*, 2nd Edition, Wadsworth, Belmont, California.

Reid, N. G. and Boore, J. R. P. (1987). *Research Methods and Statistics in Health Care*, Arnold, London.

Taylor, S. J. and Bogdan, R. (1984). *Introduction to Qualitative Research Methods: The Search for Meanings*, 2nd Edition, Wiley, New York.

Waltz, C. F., Strickland, O. L. and Lenz, E. R. (1984). *Measurement in Nursing Research*, F. A. Davis, Philadelphia.

AIMS OF THIS CHAPTER

- To examine methods of analysing data quantitatively;
- To examine methods of analysing data qualitatively;
- To explore combinations of the two approaches;
- To help select a suitable method for your project.

INTRODUCTION

In the two previous chapters we considered methods of collecting data. Often the method is tied to the type of analysis—so much so that on occasions it is difficult to separate the two. Methods of analysis must always be considered alongside data collection.

In this chapter we consider two broad approaches to data analysis:

- quantitative;
- qualitative.

Before you work through this chapter, it may be helpful to re-read the sections on the differences between quantitative and qualitative research, outlined in Chapter 4. Quantitative research tends to generate data in the form of numbers but qualitative research generates data that are made up of blocks of text that can be interpreted in various ways. The purpose of the analysis in both cases is to identify patterns or trends emerging from the data. In addition, the researcher must carry out various checks to ensure that these patterns or trends are reliable and valid. In this chapter quantitative and qualitative data analysis are discussed separately.

I TYPES OF QUANTITATIVE ANALYSIS

By the end of this section you will have discovered:

- some of the common terms used in quantitative analysis;

- some of the common tests used in quantitative analysis;
- whether any of these methods are useful to you.

Aim of the exercise To explore common terms used in quantitative analysis.

Planning stage You can do this exercise with a small group of colleagues, friends or students. Allow yourself plenty of time to complete the exercise and make notes of what you do. If you work with friends or colleagues, decide whether you will all carry out similar tasks or divide up the work between you.

Equipment/resources required Notebook, pen and access to a nursing library.

EXERCISE 8.1

What to do Work in small groups of two or three. Divide the terms listed below so that each group has two or three. Go to the library and select a range of books on research methods. Then consider the terms and write short notes on what they mean.

- statistics—descriptive and inferential
- nominal scales
- ordinal scales
- interval scales
- ratio scales
- variable
- discrete and continuous variable
- mean
- mode
- standard deviation
- normal distribution
- parametric and non-parametric tests
- median
- cumulative frequency

Write down other words that are unfamiliar to you and note down their meaning. Discuss your findings with all your colleagues. Now break into small groups again and find examples from the literature of the following ways of presenting numerical data:

- graph
- pie chart
- table
- histogram
- bar chart
- percentage component bar chart

Return to the larger group and show examples of what you found. Discuss the ways in which these methods of presentation have been used and why one method is sometimes better than another. Now decide what you need to know more about. Write a list of the items you need to study and think of ways you can gain the information.

Evaluation Discuss your findings and your progress with your colleagues and a tutor. What sort of data do you think your research project will generate? Consider how quantitative methods will help your project. Think of the advantages and disadvantages of the quantitative approach.

As another level of evaluation, it is useful, before you finish the activity, to note down:
(a) what you learned from doing the activity;
(b) how you will use what you learned;
(c) how what you have learned relates to what you have read;
(d) what you need to learn next.

INFORMATION BOX

Learning more about quantitative research

These are some routes to learning more about the subject:

evening classes at colleges and extra-mural departments of universities;

asking for a course of lectures on the topic in the school or college of nursing;

using learning packages;

working with a research supervisor;

reading;

Open University programmes on the television.

Aim of the exercise To explore some simple statistical calculations.

Planning stage This activity is best carried out by you working alone. Allow yourself plenty of time to complete the exercise and make notes of what you do.

Equipment/resources required Notebook, pen, access to a nursing library, calculator.

EXERCISE 8.2

What to do Consider the table below:

Monthly discharge rate from an acute admission psychiatric ward over two years

	Jan	Feb	Mar	Apr	May	Jun	Jul	Aug	Sep	Oct	Nov	Dec
Year 1	27	24	30	30	21	24	29	28	20	25	24	22
Year 2	29	30	26	24	20	29	30	24	22	23	23	20

Now calculate the following:

● the mean discharge rate over two years;
● the mean discharge rate for each year;
● the mean discharge rate for each month over the two-year period.

Now draw a bar chart that illustrates the mean discharge rate for each month over the two-year period. Then calculate the frequency of each of the values. Convert the data into a pie chart. Now calculate:

● the median for this set of values;
● the cumulative frequency.

If you experience any problems with these calculations, refer to:
– Reid, N. G. and Boore, J. R. P. (1987). *Research Methods and Statistics in Health Care*; Arnold, London.

Evaluation Check through your answers with a group of colleagues and with a tutor.

As another level of evaluation, it is useful, before you finish the activity, to note down:
(a) what you learned from doing the activity;
(b) how you will use what you learned;
(c) how what you have learned relates to what you have read;
(d) what you need to learn next.

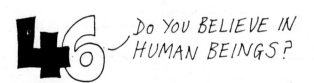 DO YOU BELIEVE IN HUMAN BEINGS?

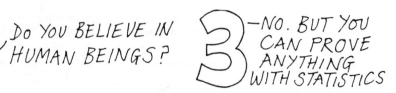 —NO. BUT YOU CAN PROVE ANYTHING WITH STATISTICS

Aim of the exercise To explore problems associated with the use of statistical arguments.

Planning stage You can do this exercise with a small group of colleagues, friends or students. Allow yourself plenty of time to complete the exercise and make notes of what you do. If you work with friends or colleagues, decide whether you will all carry out similar tasks or whether you will divide up the work between you.

Equipment/resources required Notebook, pen and access to a nursing library.

EXERCISE 8.3

What to do Read the proposition and rationale below. The rationale offers an explanation of a statistical table and the proposition is based on how the data can be interpreted. Read the passage and decide if the proposition is valid. This is an exercise in the art of reading statistics. The discussion focuses on one proposition and is divided into two parts. The first offers a statistical argument in support of the proposition. The second offers a critique of that statistical argument.

The art of reading statistics is to place them in context and to interpret them by reference to that background. This requires considerable knowledge of the relevant subject area, so read the discussions critically and carefully.

The proposition

Marriage is fatal for men

● The supporting argument

It is no longer socially unacceptable for a couple to enter into a partnership in which they live together as man and wife. This change in attitude developed from the appreciation by many adults of the real consequence of marriage—that marriage is fatal for men. The table below demonstrates this fact conclusively.

Population of England and Wales, Mid 1971 ('000s)

Age	Male	Female	Total
0–4	2 009	1 911	3 920
5–14	3 980	3 776	7 756
15–19	1 715	1 640	3 355
20–29	3 526	3 469	6 995
30–44	4 340	4 258	8 598
45–74	7 437	8 506	15 943
75 and over	713	1 534	2 247
Totals	23 720	25 094	48 814

Source: The Registrar General's *Statistical Review of England and Wales*, 1971, part 2, 1973, Table A6, 10–11.

Women outnumber men but not over all age groups. In the younger generation men outnumber women. As men grow older this situation is reversed by their death rate increasing more rapidly than the rate for women. The change occurs when men and women are in the fifth decade. Its effect is that a 3 per cent surplus of men in the younger age groups is converted to a 23 per cent surplus of women in the older age groups.

A single factor produces the change—marriage. It is sufficiently widespread to produce the change and by the time it occurs men have experienced marriage for a sufficient length of time for the change to become apparent.

● A critique of the supporting argument

The statistical argument implies that the table shows what happened over time. But the table shows the situation at a point in time—mid 1971. It therefore does not show 'a 3 per cent surplus of men in the younger age groups is converted into a 23 per cent surplus of women in the older age

continued

groups'. The only statistics which can show whether such a conversion occurs are those which compare the same group of men and women over all age groups. They are obtained by following the group throughout its life.

As an illustration of what such statistics would show consider the '75 and over' age group. It contains the largest surplus of women. Notice that a man aged 75 in 1971 would have been 20 in 1916. Clearly, the surplus of women is partly explained by deaths occurring in the First World War.

Now consider the second oldest age group. It is the only other age group in which women outnumber men. Notice that a man aged 50 in 1971 would have been 20 in 1942. Once again the surplus of women is explained partly by war deaths.

In both age groups the differences are further reduced by the residual effects of the two wars. These effects include the premature death of men who survived injury or who had been imprisoned. They also include the premature death of men who were not conscripted because of ill health.

The statistical argument states that 'a common experience . . . kills men more quickly than women'. This implies that a causal relationship exists when two factors are each experienced by a large proportion of individuals in a group. It implies that a strong statistical relationship denotes a causal relationship. A statistical relationship does nothing of the kind. All such a relationship does is show the observed strength of a causal relationship established by theory. The reason is quite simple. Statistical relationships are easy to manufacture.

As an example, suppose that in a group of ten women, eight are married and eight wear jeans. At least six (75 per cent) of the married women wear jeans. Consequently there is a strong statistical relationship between being married and wearing jeans. As this is a fabricated relationship, it is quite meaningless, despite its apparent strength. If this were not so, the relationship would show that only married women normally wear jeans. In this case the converse would also be true—that single women do not normally wear jeans. We know that neither is true.

Clearly, the statistical argument about marriage and death is defective. The comparison should be between married men and women, not all men and women. The measure of the effect of marriage should be the length of marriage at death, not the age of the individual.

Individually the deficiencies raise doubts about the validity of the statistical argument. Together they establish that it is totally unsound. The statistical argument therefore does not support the proposition. It does not establish that marriage is fatal for men.

Evaluation Now evaluate the proposition. Can you spot any problems in the arguments? Do not give up too quickly. The development of critical skills is an important one. Do you agree with the critique? Can you identify any problems not spotted by the critique? Is the critique fair?

As another level of evaluation, it is useful, before you finish the activity, to note down:

(a) what you learned from doing the activity;
(b) how you will use what you learned;
(c) how what you have learned relates to what you have read;
(d) what you need to learn next.

This exercise is based on work by Mr Bunny le Roux, Principal Lecturer, Department of Applied Statistics and Operational Research, Sheffield City Polytechnic and is reproduced with permission.

2 EXPLORING QUALITATIVE ANALYSIS

By the end of this section you will have discovered:

● how to identify different frameworks for analysing qualitative data;
● whether or not any of these methods are useful.

Aim of the exercise To explore qualitative analysis of data.

Planning stage You can do this exercise with a small group of colleagues, friends or students. Allow yourself plenty of time to complete the exercise and make notes of what you do. If you work with friends or colleagues, decide whether you will all carry out similar tasks or whether you will divide up the work between you.

Equipment/resources required Notebook, pen and access to a nursing library.

EXERCISE 8.4

What to do Read through the following extract from an interview with a patient. The interview comes from a study of patients' perceptions of the information they have been given about their illness. As you read through, consider what sorts of statements the person is making and whether or not a number of them fall into groups.

'I've been on the ward about six weeks now ... no one really tells you very much ... I mean, the doctor talked to my husband and my daughter. He didn't talk to me. I get very depressed about it all. Sometimes I don't sleep all that well. Mind you, I don't sleep very well at home, either. The sister's very good. She always answers any questions I have but she doesn't seem to want to talk to me about what's wrong with me .... I think I know though. My daughter always tells me not to worry. I get scared sometimes. Why won't they tell me?

'I go to physiotherapy twice a week. Susan, down there, always says how well I'm doing. I don't think she really knows the whole story. She's more interested in my leg! I like it down there, though ... I meet a lot of other people. You can talk to other people because they're in the same boat. I don't get so fed up down there. It's the company, I think. Mind you, my husband tries to talk to me. It's not the same in hospital, though.'

The aim of a qualitative analysis of this sort of data is to classify as many statements or units of meaning as possible from the data so that the researcher can make sense of it. The generation of categories of response also allows for comparisons to be made between different sets of data.

Read through the passage above again and try to organise phrases under the following headings:

● types of people discussed;
● feelings expressed;
● activities;
● levels of communication;
● comments about being in hospital;
● comparisons of hospital life with other aspects of life;
● theories about communication in hospital;
● comments about illness.

Now read the material listed below and compare the method you have just explored with others qualitative methods.

– Hycner, R. H. (1985). Some Guidelines for the Phenomenological Analysis of Interview Data; *Human Studies*, 8, 279–303.
– Melia, K. M. (1987). *Learning and Working: The Occupational Socialisation of Nurses*; Tavistock, London.
– Watson, J. (1985). *Nursing: Human Science and Human Care: A Theory of Nursing*; Appleton-Century-Crofts, Norwalk, Connecticut.

continued

Evaluation Discuss your category system with your colleagues. Consider whether your method would be a useful way to analyse your data.

As another level of evaluation, it is useful, before you finish the activity, to note down:
(a) what you learned from doing the activity;
(b) how you will use what you learned;
(c) how what you have learned relates to what you have read;
(d) what you need to learn next.

CONCLUSION

You have now explored two approaches to handling data. From a philosophical point of view, the quantitative and qualitative approaches start from very different assumptions about the nature of research. From a practical point of view, it is possible to use and combine both approaches. For a further discussion of this combined approach, read:
– Bryman, A. (1988). *Quantity and Quality in Social Research*; Unwin Hyman, London.

LEARNING CHECK

If you are a working on your own
● Read through the notes you have made while completing the exercises in this chapter and consider the following questions:
– What new knowledge have I gained?
– What new skills have I developed?
– How has my thinking about research changed?
– What do I need to do now?
● Check that you have made reference cards for any new references that you have found whilst working on the exercises in this chapter.

If you are working in a small group
● Pair off and nominate one of you as A and one of you as B. For five minutes, A talks to B about what has been learned and B listens. This should not be a conversation: B's only role is to listen. After five minutes, roles are reversed and B talks to A about what has been learned and A listens. After the second five minutes, re-form into a group and discuss the experience.

If you are a tutor and/or facilitator
● Use the above 'pairs' exercise with the group you are working with.
● Hold two 'rounds' in which each person in turn says what was liked *least* about doing the activities and what was liked *most* about doing the activities.

9 · UNDERTAKING THE RESEARCH PROJECT

WHAT YOU NEED TO READ

Armitage, S. and Rees, C. (1988). Student Projects, a Practical Framework, *Nurse Education Today*, 8, 289–295.

British Psychological Society (1987). Code of Practice on Supervision, Preparation and Examination of Doctoral Theses in Departments of Psychology, *Bulletin of the British Psychological Society*, 40, 250–254.

Hawthorne, P. J. (1981). Supervision of Dissertations of Undergraduate Nursing Students, *Nursing Times*, 77, 8, 29–30.

Howard, K. and Sharp, J. A. (1983). *The Management of a Student Research Project*, Gower, Aldershot.

Mander, R. (1988). Encouraging Students to be Research Minded, *Nurse Education Today*, 8, 30–35.

AIMS OF THIS CHAPTER

- To enable you to structure your time;
- To consider aspects of supervision;
- To plan and work consistently through your project.

INTRODUCTION

All the previous chapters have focused on discrete parts of the research process. Our aim in this chapter is to pull the threads together to enable you to work through the project as a whole.

I TIME MANAGEMENT

By the end of this section you will have discovered:

- how to plan your work;
- how to use time effectively.

Aim of the exercise To plan your research project in terms of time.

Planning stages This exercise should be carried out in a small group. Allow yourself plenty of time to complete the exercise and make notes of what you do. If you work with friends or colleagues, decide whether you will all carry out similar tasks or divide up the work between you.

Equipment/resources required Notebook, pen and access to a nursing library.

EXERCISE 9.1

What to do You are going to use the process known as 'outlining'. First, jot down the broad stages of your research project. These may include:

- planning;
- searching the literature;
- collecting data;
- analysing data;
- writing.

Now think about the time you will have available for each stage and write that next to each heading. Then take each of these stages in turn and write down the individual tasks that have to be completed for each of them. Write down the amount of time each task will require. When you have completed each stage, see if you can cut back on any tasks. It is useful if you consider your planning under the following three headings:

- what *must* be done;
- what *should* be done;
- what *could* be done.

After you have completed this job draw up a 'master plan' of your research project showing how aspects of your work will fit into a time scale. Some tasks will run concurrently with others.

Evaluation Discuss your plan with your supervisor and with your colleagues. Ask them to look for problems in your planning. An organised approach will help your project to run smoothly.

As another level of evaluation, it is useful, before you finish the activity, to note down:
(a) what you learned from doing the activity;
(b) how you will use what you learned;
(c) how what you have learned relates to what you have read;
(d) what you need to learn next.

INFORMATION BOX

Aspects of time management

keep detailed notes as you progress through your project;

discipline your approach;

keep detailed reference cards up to date;

be systematic;

keep in touch with your supervisor;

don't leave everything to the last minute;

don't expect your supervisor to do your project for you;

don't expect your supervisor to see you without an appointment;

don't expect your local library to have all the references you require.

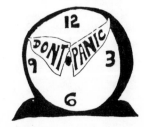

2 SUPERVISION OF YOUR RESEARCH PROJECT

A supervisor is the person who oversees your research project. The job is usually performed by a tutor or lecturer in the department in which you are studying. Supervisors have usually completed research of their own and may be working on new projects.

By the end of this section you will have discovered:

● what you can expect of your supervisor;
● what your supervisor can expect of you.

Aim of the exercise To explore the role of the supervisor.

Planning stage This exercise should be carried out on your own and then your findings discussed in a small group. Allow yourself plenty of time to complete the exercise and make notes of what you do.

Equipment/resources required Notebook, pen and access to a nursing library.

EXERCISE 9.2

What to do Sit down and write out a list entitled 'What I expect from a supervisor'. Now ask your supervisor to undertake a similar exercise, writing two lists—'What I can offer as a supervisor' and 'What I expect from my students'.

Evaluation When you have carried out these two tasks, sit and discuss your roles and negotiate a working relationship for the research project.

As another level of evaluation, it is useful, before you finish the activity, to note down:
(a) what you learned from doing the activity;
(b) how you will use what you learned;
(c) how what you have learned relates to what you have read;
(d) what you need to learn next.

INFORMATION BOX

A checklist for achieving good research supervision

Completing a project is a joint venture involving a student and a supervisor. Here are some items which can help promote good supervisory practice.

Several of these items are adapted from the guidelines provided by the Science and Engineering Research Council (1983).

Supervisor

what steps have been taken to try and make a good match between a supervisor and the student?

does the supervisor allocate adequate time to meet the student?

does the supervisor insist on written material throughout the project?

does the supervisor insist on setting aims for the next meeting?

has the supervisor demonstrated how to make systematic records?

does the supervisor help the student to select problems, stimulate and motivate the student and provide a steady stream of scientific ideas and guidance?

Student

have you planned your project satisfactorily?

have you identified key problem areas?

do you understand the relevant literature?

do you keep accurate and systematic records of what you read and what you do?

do you write your project as you progress from stage to stage?

do you approach your supervisor for help, giving adequate time for an appointment to be made and, where appropriate, specifying the problem?

CONCLUSION

In this book we have tried to show that *you* can do research. The main theme running through this particular chapter has been the need for a planned and systematic approach. While research is not easy, it is simpler if you plan it properly. The need to be systematic is part of the research process itself. You cannot claim validity for your project if you cannot account for certain aspects of it.

The systematic approach needs to be sustained. The systematic approach will help you to keep going when you are less enthusiastic.

An efficient researcher will think in terms of 'sub goals'. A sense of achievement will be reinforced by having achieved each of these smaller tasks. On the other hand, if you do not break down tasks in this way, you may find yourself daunted by the size of the work.

LEARNING CHECK

If you are working on your own
- Read through the notes you made while completing the exercises in this chapter and consider the following questions:
  - What new knowledge have I gained?
  - What new skills have I developed?
  - How has my thinking about research changed?
  - What do I need to do now?
- Check that you have made reference cards for any new references that you have found whilst working on the exercises in this chapter.

If you are working in a small group
- Pair off and nominate one of you as A and one of you as B. For five minutes, A talks to B about what has been learned and B listens. This should not be a conversation: B's only role is to listen. After five minutes, roles are reversed and B talks to A about what has been learned and A listens. After the second five minutes, re-form into a group and discuss the experience.

If you are a tutor and/or facilitator
- Use the above 'pairs' exercise with the group you are working with.
- Hold two 'rounds' in which each person in turn says what was liked *least* about doing the activities and what was liked *most* about doing the activities.

10 · WRITING THE RESEARCH REPORT

WHAT YOU NEED TO READ

Barzun, J. and Graff, H. E. (1977). *The Modern Researcher*, 3rd Edition, Harcourt, Brace Jovanovich, New York.

Bell, J. (1987). Writing the Report; in Bell, J. *Doing Your Research Project: A Guide for First-Time Researchers in Education and Social Science*, Open University Press, Milton Keynes; p. 124–135.

Bogdan, R. C. and Biklen, S. K. (1982). *Qualitative Research for Education: An Introduction to Theory and Methods*, Allyn and Bacon, Boston, Mass.

Morris, S. (1988). Writing a Book: Some Advice for New Authors, *Nurse Education Today*, 8, 234–238.

AIMS OF THIS CHAPTER

● To identify the stages in writing a research report;
● To consider how to submit a research report to a journal;
● To feed back your findings to the participants in your study.

INTRODUCTION

All research has to be recorded to demonstrate how you have carried out your work and how you reached your conclusions. A research report allows you to share your findings with others and adds to the body of knowledge in a particular subject. You may also want to have your research report considered for publication in a nursing magazine or journal. In this way, your work reaches a wider audience.

1 PLANNING YOUR RESEARCH REPORT

By the end of this section you will have discovered:

● the structure of a research report;
● how to write in an orderly way;
● how to write for publication.

EXERCISE 10.1

Aim of the exercise To explore various ways of structuring a research report.

Planning stage You can do this exercise on your own or in the company of a small group of colleagues, friends or students. Allow yourself plenty of time to complete the exercise and make notes of what you do. If you work with friends or colleagues, decide whether you will all carry out similar tasks or whether you will divide up the work between you.

Equipment/resources required Notebook, pen and access to a nursing library.

What to do Go to the library and study the research reports listed below. Make notes about the headings each writer uses, the degree to which illustrations and tables aid clarity, and the differences between handling quantitative and qualitative data. Then decide the style of writing which would suit your work and the skills you need to develop to write your report.

The studies to review are:

– Bogdan, R., Brown, M. A. and Foster, S. B. (1982). Be Honest But Not Cruel: Staff/Patient Communication on a Neonatal Unit; *Human Organisation*, 41, 1, 6–16.
– Burnard, P. and Morrison, P. (1988). Nurses' Perceptions of Their Interpersonal Skills: a Descriptive Study Using Six Category Intervention Analysis; *Nurse Education Today*, 8, 266–272.
– Melia, K. M. (1987). *Learning and Working: The Occupational Socialisation of Nurses*; Tavistock, London.
– Morrison, P. and le Roux, B. (1987). The Practice of Seclusion; *Nursing Times*, 83, 19, 62–66.

Evaluation Discuss your findings with your colleagues and decide what skills you each possess or lack.

As another level of evaluation, it is useful, before you finish the activity, to note down:

(a) what you learned from doing the activity;
(b) how you will use what you learned;
(c) how what you have learned relates to what you have read;
(d) what you need to learn next.

INFORMATION BOX

Structuring research reports

There is no right way to structure a research report. However, certain headings and sub-headings are common. If you have been logical in your research your report will also be orderly. Headings that you may want to consider are:

Title
Summary
Aims
Rationale
Review of the literature
Methods used

Results
Analysis and discussion of results
Conclusions and recommendations
References
Appendices.

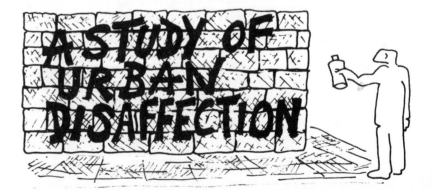

2 WRITING YOUR REPORT

By the end of this section you will have discovered:

● how to write clearly;
● the materials needed for writing a report;
● how to present your report.

Aim of the exercise To explore approaches to writing a research report.

Planning stage You can do this exercise on your own or in the company of a small group of colleagues, friends or students. Allow yourself plenty of time to complete the exercise and make notes of what you do. If you work with friends or colleagues, decide whether you will all carry out similar tasks or whether you will divide up the work between you.

Equipment/resources required Notebook, pen and access to a nursing library.

EXERCISE 10.2

What to do Look at a selection of student dissertations and theses. If you cannot find them try getting some through the Inter-Library Loan system. The publications to choose from are:

– Barker, P. (1988). Nursing the Patient With Major Affective Disorder; PhD Thesis, Dundee College of Technology.
– Elkind, A. K. (1980). Smoking Amongst Women with Special Reference to those Training for a Profession; PhD Thesis, University of Manchester.
– Fretwell, J. F. (1979). Socialisation of Nurses: Teaching and Learning in Hospital Wards; PhD Thesis, University of Warwick.
– Moyes, B. (1976). Perceptions of Pregnancy; PhD Thesis, University of Edinburgh.
– Muir-Cochrane, E. (1983). An examination of the psychiatric nursing component of degree/SRN courses at Universities and Polytechnics in England, Scotland and Wales; BN Dissertation, Chelsea College, University of London.

As you look through these reports make notes on:

● the binding;
● the table of contents;
● the size of margins;
● the page numbering system;
● how words are laid out on the page;
● the headings used;
● the existence of appendices;
● the presentation of references.

Find out if there are rules about the presentation of your report specified by your college or school.

Bear in mind that the reports you have looked at are submitted for higher degrees. The reports therefore offer good examples of layout and presentation.

Evaluation Discuss you findings with your colleagues and write a list of items you need to consider about layout and style for your research report.

As another level of evaluation, it is useful, before you finish the activity, to note down:
(a) what you learned from doing the activity;
(b) how you will use what you learned;
(c) how what you have learned relates to what you have read;
(d) what you need to learn next.

INFORMATION BOX

Writing clearly

use short sentences;

do not use long words instead of short ones;

keep jargon and technical terms to a minimum;

do not use long paragraphs;

use headings to guide readers;

edit your work frequently;

be prepared to make several drafts of your report;

show your work to your supervisor for comment;

if necessary, consult a style manual. Suitable style manuals include:
– *CBE Style Manual*; 5th Edition, Council of Biology Editors, Bethesda, Maryland.
– Gowers, E. (revised by B. Fraser) (1977). *The Complete Plain Words*; 2nd Edition, Penguin, London.
– Strunk, W. Jr. and White, E. B. (1972). *The Elements of Style*; 2nd Edition, Macmillan, New York.
– Turabian, K. L. (1973). *A Manual For Writers of Term Papers, Theses and Dissertations*; 4th Edition, University of Chicago Press, Chicago.

3 WRITING FOR PUBLICATION

By the end of this section you will have discovered:

● how to prepare your work for publication;
● how to get guidelines for publication.

INFORMATION BOX

Opportunities for publication

Your report could be considered for publication by a number of organisations. Some opportunities for publishing your work include:

a journal

a chapter in a book

a book

a monograph published by your college

a conference paper.

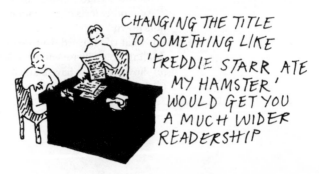

CHANGING THE TITLE TO SOMETHING LIKE 'FREDDIE STARR ATE MY HAMSTER' WOULD GET YOU A MUCH WIDER READERSHIP

EXERCISE 10.3

Aim of the exercise To explore material on research report writing.

Planning stage You can do this exercise on your own or in the company of a small group of colleagues, friends or students. Allow yourself plenty of time to complete the exercise and make notes of what you do. If you work with friends or colleagues, decide whether you will all carry out similar tasks or whether you will divide up the work between you.

Equipment/resources required Notebook, pen and access to a nursing library.

What to do Obtain the books listed below, from the library. Read them and make notes under the following headings: interest, relevance, style, appeal.
Now study the following books on writing for publication:
– O'Connor, M. (1978). *Editing Scientific Books and Journals*; Pitman Medical, London.
– Starr, A. D. (1988). *Science Writing for Beginners*; Blackwell, Oxford.
– Sternberg, R. J. (1988). *The Psychologist's Companion: A Guide to Writing Scientific Writing for Students and Researchers*; Cambridge University Press, Cambridge.

Evaluation Discuss your findings with your colleagues and list the constituents of a good report. Remember that, from the publishers' point of view, the main question is 'can this be published?' This raises different evaluation criteria than those which apply to evaluating research reports that are not for publication.

As another level of evaluation, it is useful, before you finish the activity, the note down:
(a) what you learned from doing the activity;
(b) how you will use what you learned;
(c) how what you have learned relates to what you have read;
(d) what you need to learn next.

INFORMATION BOX
Submitting work for publication

Getting your report published may be important to spread knowledge. However, you may have to wait some time before you see your work published and there is no guarantee that your work will be accepted. To speed up the process:

approach one journal with the idea of your report;

only submit an article to one journal at a time;

ask editors for a guide to their house style (*Advice to Authors*);

submit clean copies.

Always be prepared for a journal to reject your work. Some may write back with details of how your work could be modified. If you do get advice on how to revise your work, follow that advice carefully.

CONCLUSION

You have now completed your research! Now you can consider your next move: will you do more research, further study or perhaps another course? Your work has stopped for the moment but if you are to continue your education you need to consider the next step. We hope that you have enjoyed working through this book and through the process of research.

LEARNING CHECK

If you are a working on your own
- Read through the notes you made while completing the exercises in this chapter and consider the following questions:
  - What new knowledge have I gained?
  - What new skills have I developed?
  - How has my thinking about research changed?
  - What do I need to do now?
- Check that you have made reference cards for any new references that you have found whilst working on the exercises in this chapter.

If you are working in a small group
- Pair off and nominate one of you as A and one of you as B. For five minutes, A talks to B about what has been learned and B listens. This should be a conversation: B's only role is to listen. After five minutes, roles are reversed and B talks to A about what has been learned and A listens. After the second five minutes, re-form into a group and discuss the experience.

If you are a tutor and/or facilitator
- Use the above 'pairs' exercise with the group you are working with.
- Hold two 'rounds' in which each person in turn says what was liked *least* about doing the activities and what was liked *most* about doing the activities.

◆COMPENDIUM OF USEFUL INFORMATION

In this compendium you will find a whole host of ideas and pointers to
further information which will help any nurse involved in research.
The compendium does not pretend to be exhaustive but it does point
you in the right direction for a successful project.

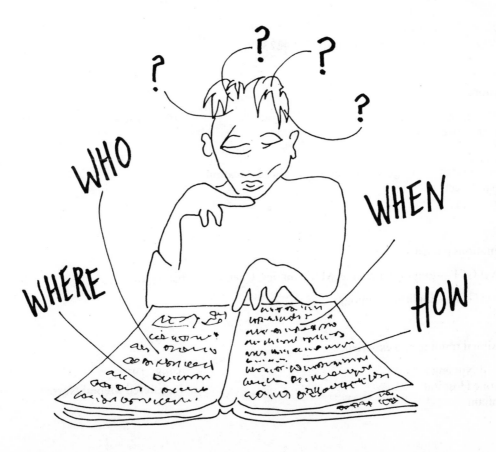

1 A SAMPLE CURRICULUM VITAE

Personal details

John Davies
21 Dyserth Drive
Cardiff
South Glamorgan
CF6 8ET

Telephone: Cardiff (0222) 23245

Nationality: British

Age: 40

Married with two children

Date of Birth: 18 April 1948

Occupation: Nurse tutor

Work Address: School of Nursing Studies
South Glamorgan School of Nursing
South Glamorgan General Hospital
East Park
Cardiff
CF5 6TG
Telephone: Cardiff (0222) 422379

Education

Cardiff Central High School 3 Ascroft Grove Cardiff	1959–1964
South Glamorgan College of Further and Higher Education 18 Broad Street Cardiff	1966

Examinations passed

'O' Level GCE—English Language, Mathematics, Chemistry, History and Art.

'A' Level GCE—English, Sociology.

Professional training and experience

School of Nursing Hamstone Hospital Beckenham Kent	1968–1971 Registered Mental Nurse

School of Nursing Reedham General Hospital Croydon Surrey		1971–1973 State Registered Nurse
West Hampstead College of Higher Education Banker's Park Hampstead		1974–1976 Diploma in Nursing
Glanville College Cheam Surrey		1980–1981 Certificate of Education

Awarded Registered Nurse Teacher Certificate in 1981

Posts held

Nurse tutor	1981–present	School of Nursing Studies South Glamorgan School of Nursing South Glamorgan General Hospital East Park Cardiff CF5 6TG
Charge nurse	1979–1981	Mid Glamorgan Hospital Cuthbert Place Caerphilly Mid Glamorgan
Staff nurse	1976–1979	Mid Glamorgan Hospital
Staff nurse	1973–1976	School of Nursing Reedham General Hospital Croydon Surrey

Outline of responsibilities

I am a psychiatric nurse tutor responsible for planning and implementing the 1982 Syllabus of Training for psychiatric nursing students. I am also personal tutor to 24 students and I have organised and run a small staff support group in the acute services area.

I have responsibility for helping to set and mark final examinations papers and I am an Assessor for the English National Board for Nursing, Midwifery and Health Visiting.

Professional courses attended

Assessors Course	1982	Crowham Hospital Mardy Mid Glamorgan
Experiential Learning Methods Course	1983	Department of Educational Studies University of Wales Extra Mural Department Forest Place

Publication

Davies, J. (1984) Learning to Teach Interpersonal Skills: *Nurse Educational Journal*; 3, 4, 22–28.

Hobbies and interests

Swimming, reading, collecting butterflies, family life.

Other details

Full Driving Licence
Chairman of the Mid Glamorgan Nursing Research Interest Group

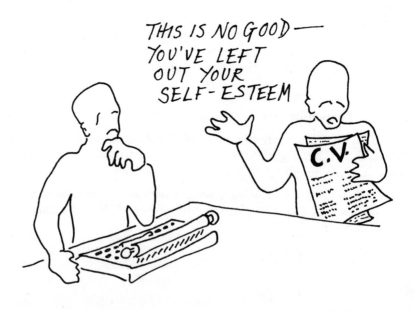

THIS IS NO GOOD —
YOU'VE LEFT
OUT YOUR
SELF-ESTEEM

2 HOW TO QUOTE REFERENCES IN RESEARCH REPORTS

Clear and accurate references should always be offered in a research report. These references allow other readers to:

- verify what you write;
- develop your ideas further;
- identify other sources of reading.

It is important that you only list publications that you have actually read so that your use of references is accurate. It is also important that you record your references accurately and systematically. Various methods of referencing are available but perhaps the most frequently used method is known as the Harvard method.

Attention to the details of this system is important and it is vital that you do not mix two sorts of referencing systems together! Learn this one and use it accurately. Once learned, the method of referencing can be used for nearly all essays, papers and submissions to journals.

THE HARVARD REFERENCING SYSTEM

In the text you refer to references by surname only and year of publication, as illustrated in the following passage.

> *Although first prepared by Benedikt (1879), its structure was not confirmed until much later (Osborn and Jay, 1955). Fox, Keenan and Trueside (1983) have recently shown that it is a good chlorinating agent.*

Note that when you reference in this way, you do not refer to the title of the book or article in the text. This is listed in a separate section of your report.

If you quote directly from a reference and you only want to quote a few words, you do so as follows:

> *Counselling has been described as the process of 'exploring the other person's world' (Black 1986).*

If you quote direct from a reference and you want to quote a slightly longer piece, you do so as follows:

> *'Empathy is the intimate process of coming to view the world as the other person views it: to enter into the other person's frame of reference' (Black, 1986, 22–3).*

If you want to use a quotation that has already been used by another writer, you do so as follows:

> *'Empathy cannot be taught, it can only be learned through direct personal experience' (Brown, cited by White, 1987, p. 22).*

In the reference list, you then list *White's* book—the one that contained the quotation. Wherever possible, you should avoid quoting from secondary sources. Try to go back to the original.

If you want to quote from a chapter, by one author, that is contained in a book edited by another, you do so as follows:

> *Interpersonal skills may be taught in a variety of settings. As one writer points out: 'Interpersonal skills training is often associated with psychiatric nursing. It is just as vital in general nursing, health visiting and district nursing.' (Jones, 1987, p. 34)*

In the reference list, the chapter is entered as follows:

> Jones, D. (1987). Teaching Interpersonal Skills, in D. Brown (ed), A Handbook of Training Methods for Nurses, Heinemann, London.

Note, particularly, the style of layout of this reference and the underlining procedure. For further details of this, see below.

There are certain specific points to be made about using direct quotes:

● only use quotations that add significantly to your work;
● when you use a direct quotation, keep it short and indent the paragraph;
● after the quotation and in brackets, identify the author, date of publication and page number(s).

At the end of your paper you should include a list of references. This should be in alphabetical order of authors' surnames and is subject to certain conventions. If you are referencing a book in your list, it should appear as in the following example:

> Burnard, P. (1985). Learning Human Skills: A Guide for Nurses, Heinemann, London.

A book is identified by the following details:

● author;
● date of publication;
● title;
● publisher;
● place of publication.

If you are referencing a journal article it should appear as follows:

> Riebel, L. (1984). A Homeopathic Model of Psychotherapy; Journal of Humanistic Psychology, vol 24, No. 2, 9–14.

A journal article is identified by the following details:

● author;
● date of publication;
● title of the article;
● name of the journal;
● volume number;
● edition number;
● page range.

Note an important difference between referencing books and articles. In the case of a book, the title is underlined, but in the case of an article, the name of the *journal* is underlined.

Reference lists differ from bibliographies, which provide a further list of books and journals that the writer has found of interest. Normally, a research report will contain only a reference list.

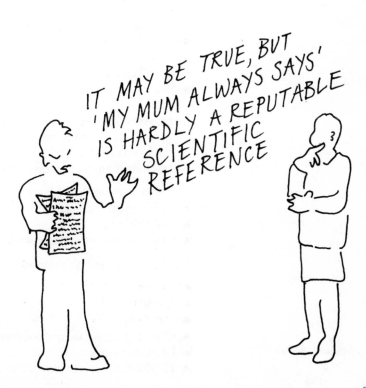

3 COMPUTER PROGRAMS

Computer programs are always being improved. This list offers an idea of the range of programs available.

Computer programs fall into categories:

● word processing;
● databases;
● spreadsheets;
● integrated programs;
● statistical programs.

Word processors are the programs that help you to write your report. A good word-processing package will include many of the following facilities:

● word counting;
● spelling check;
● movement of text;
● ability to edit two documents concurrently;
● fast movement through text.

Examples of word processing programs are:

● First Word Plus;
● Manuscript;
● Microsoft Word;
● Protext;
● Total Word;
● Volkswriter;
● WordPerfect;
● WordStar.

Databases allow you to store information. You may use such a program to store all the references that you collect or to store the research data that you have accumulated. A good database program will include many of the following facilities:

● fast movement through entries;
● alphabetical sorting;
● flexibility;
● ability to import and export data.

Examples of database programs are:

● Aspect;
● Cardbox;
● Dataflex;
● dBase;
● Paradox;
● PC File.

Spreadsheets allow you to draw large 'grids' and tables to allow you to think about and analyse your data. A good spreadsheet program will include many of the following facilities:

- flexibility;
- ability to import data;
- simple word processing;
- mathematical and statistical ability;
- graphics.

Examples of spreadsheet programs are:

- Lotus 1–2–3;
- PlanPerfect;
- SuperCalc;
- Swift;
- VP Planner;
- Words and Figures.

Integrated programs incorporate word processing, database and spreadsheet functions. An integrated program allows you to transfer data quickly from one element of the program to another. The drawbacks of such programs are that they are often expensive to buy and the individual elements of the program may not be so easy to use as separate programs. A good integrated program will include many of the following facilities:

- easy transfer of data;
- ease of use;
- good graphics.

Examples of integrated programs are:

- Ability;
- Able One;
- Enable;
- Framework;
- Smart;
- Symphony.

Statistical packages are those programs that help you with the analysis of data. Many spreadsheet programs are also able to do statistical calculations.

Examples of statistical packages are:

- Amstat;
- Forecasting;
- Oxystat;
- Resource Management.

Other programs are available to help you prepare, analyse and present your data. Programs that you may want to consider are those concerned with:

- analysing data;
- creating an index;
- creating graphics;
- desktop publishing;
- expert systems;
- money management;
- teaching.

Useful introductory texts for computing include:
- Billings, D. M. (1986). *Computer Assisted Instruction for Health Professionals: A Guide to Designing and Using CAL*; Appleton-Century-Crofts, Norwalk, Connecticut.
- Blease, D. (1986). *Evaluating Educational Software*; Croom Helm, London.
- Gosling, P. E. (1982). *Mastering Computer Programming*; Macmillan, London.
- Hartley, P. J. (1976). *Introduction to BASIC: a Case Study Approach*; Macmillan, London.
- O'Neil, P. (1981). *Computer-Based Instruction*; Academic Press, New York.
- Procter, P. (1988). *Nurses and Computers*; Croom Helm, London.
- Rowntree, G. (ed) (1987). *Fundamentals of Computing*; NCC Publications, Manchester.
- Sanderson, P. C. (1980). *An Introduction to Microcomputer Programming*; Butterworth, London.

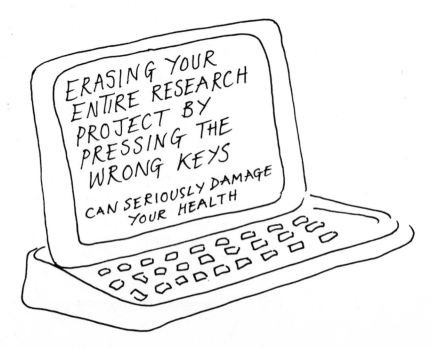

4 LITERATURE RESOURCES

It is important that your literature search is as comprehensive as possible. Here is a list of possible sources of information.

Books	Colleagues	Leaflets
Journals	Computer searches	Unpublished reports
Papers	Supervisors	Posters
Special libraries	Radio or TV	Handouts
RCN	Teletext	People from other disciplines
DSS	Reports	

5 ETHICAL CODES

Ethical issues frequently arise when conducting research. One way of thinking about ethical dilemmas is to consult a code of conduct. In 1984, the United Kingdom Central Council for Nursing, Midwifery and Health Visiting produced the following Code of Professional Conduct.

Each registered nurse, midwife and health visitor shall act, at all times, in such a manner as to justify public trust and confidence, to uphold and enhance the good standing and reputation of the profession, to serve the interests of society, and above all to safeguard the interests of individual patients and clients.

Each registered nurse, midwife and health visitor is accountable for his or her practice and, in the exercise of professional accountability shall:

1 Act always in such a way as to promote and safeguard the well being and interests of patients/clients.

2 Ensure that no action or omission on his/her part or within his/her sphere of influence is detrimental to the condition of safety of patients/clients.

3 Take every reasonable opportunity to maintain professional knowledge and competence.

4 Acknowledge any limitations of competence and refuse in such cases to accept delegated functions without first having received instruction in regard to those functions and having been assessed as competent.

5 Work in a collaborative and co-operative manner with other health care professionals and recognise and respect their particular contributions within the health care team.

6 Take account of the customs, values and spiritual beliefs of patients/clients.

7 Make known to an appropriate person or authority any conscientious objections which may be relevant to professional practice.

8 Avoid any abuse of privileged relationship which exists with patients/clients and of the privileged access allowed to their property, residence or workman.

9 Respect confidential information obtained in the course of professional practice and refrain from disclosing such information without the consent of the patient/client, or a person entitled to act on his/her behalf, except where disclosure is required by law or by the order of a court or is necessary in the public interest.

10 Have regard to the environment of care and its physical, psychological and social effects on patients/clients, and also to the adequacy of resources, and make known to appropriate persons or

authorities any circumstances which could place patients/clients in jeopardy or which militate against safe standards of practice.

11 Have regard to the workload of and the pressures on professional colleagues and subordinates and take appropriate action if these are seen to be such to constitute abuse of the individual practitioner and/or to jeopardise safe standards of practice.

12 In the context of the individual's own knowledge, experience, and sphere of authority, assist peers and subordinates to develop professional competence in accordance with their needs.

13 Refuse to accept any gift, favour or hospitality which might be interpreted as seeking to exert undue influence to obtain preferential consideration.

14 Avoid the use of professional qualifications in the promotion of commercial products in order not to compromise the independence of professional judgement on which patients/clients rely.

Nurses, too, are often required to take into account medical decisions when planning their research. In 1964, guidelines for doctors working in clinical research were laid down by the World Medical Assembly. The Declaration of Helsinki reads as follows:

> In the treatment of the sick person, the doctor must be free to use a new therapeutic measure if, in his judgment, it offers hope of saving life, re-establishing health, or alleviating suffering.
>
> If at all possible, consistent with patient psychology, the doctor should obtain the patient's freely given consent after the patient has been given a full explanation. In case of legal incapacity, consent should be procured from the legal guardian; in case of physical incapacity, the permission of the legal guardian replaces that of the patient.
>
> The doctor can combine clinical research with professional care, the objective being the acquisition of new medical knowledge, only to the extent that clinical research is justified by its therapeutic value for the patient.
>
> In the purely scientific application of clinical research carried out on a human being, it is the duty of the doctor to remain the protector of life and health of that person on whom clinical research is being carried out.
>
> The nature, the purpose, and the risk of clinical research must be explained to the subject by the doctor.
>
> Clinical research on a human being cannot be undertaken without his free consent, after he has been fully informed; if he is legally incompetent, the consent of the legal guardian should be procured.
>
> The subject of clinical research should be in such a mental, physical and legal state as to be able to exercise fully his power of choice.

Consent should, as a rule, be obtained in writing. However, the responsibility for clinical research always remains with the research worker; it never falls on the subject even after consent is obtained.

The investigator must respect the right of each individual to safeguard his personal integrity, especially if the subject is in a dependent relationship to the investigator.

At any time during the course of clinical research, the subject or his guardian should be free to withdraw permission for research to be continued. The investigator or the investigating team should discontinue the research if, in his or their judgment it may, if continued, be harmful to the individual.

References

— UKCC (1984). *Code of Professional Conduct for the Nurse, Midwife and Health Visitor*; 2nd Edition, United Kingdom Central Council for Nursing, Midwifery and Health Visiting, London.
— Declaration of Helsinki: *Recommendations Guiding Doctors in Clinical Research, Adopted by the 18th World Medical Assembly, Helsinki, Finland, 1964.*
— RCN (1977). *Ethics Related to Research in Nursing*; Royal College of Nursing, London.

6 LIST OF NURSING JOURNALS

Nursing Times
Nursing Standard
Nurse Education Today
Journal of Advanced Nursing
The Professional Nurse
International Journal of Nursing Studies
Advances in Nursing Science
Nursing Research
Nursing Outlook
Western Journal of Nursing Research
Scholarly Inquiry for Nursing Practice
The Journal of Gerontological Nursing
Health Visitor
Nursing, the add-on Journal

Journal of District Nursing
Nursing Clinics of North America
American Journal of Nursing
Archives of Psychiatric Nursing
Research in Nursing and Health
Advances in Nursing Science
Journal of Nursing Education
Journal of Obstetrics, Gynaecological and Neonatal Nursing
Journal of Psychiatric Nursing and Mental Health Services
Nursing Administration Quarterly
Maternal-Child Nursing Journal
Research in Nursing and Health

7 LISTS OF BIBLIOGRAPHIES, INDEXES AND ABSTRACTS

Nursing Bibliography, RCN

International Nursing Index, National Library of Medicine

Hospital Abstracts, HMSO

Social Services Abstracts, DSS

Current Literature on Health Services, DOH

Nursing Research Abstracts, DOH

British National Bibliography, British Library Bibliographic Services Division

Subject Guide to Books in Print, Bowker

British Books in Print, Whitaker

Bibliographic Index, Wilson

The British Education Index, British Library Services Division

Education Index, Wilson

Current Index to Journals in Education, Macmillan

British Humanities Index, Wilson

The Social Science/Humanities Indexes, Wilson

Social Sciences Citation Index, Institute for Scientific Information

Resources in Education, ERIC

Current Index to Journals in Education, ERIC

Sociology of Education Abstracts, Information for Education

Research into Higher Education, Society for Research into Higher Education

Technical Education Abstracts, Information for Education

Child Development Abstracts and Bibliography, University of Chicago Press

Psychological Abstracts, American Psychological Association

Index to Theses, ASLIB

Catalogue of Government Publication, HMSO

Social Trends, HMSO

8 TESTS, SCALES AND OTHER INSTRUMENTS FOR DATA COLLECTION

Andrulis, R. A. (1977). *A Source Book of Tests and Measures of Human Behaviour*; Charles C. Thomas, Springfield, Illinois.

Beere, C. A. (1979). *Women and Women's Issues: A Handbook of Tests and Measurements*; Jossey Bass, San Francisco, California.

Bonjean, C. M., Hill, R. J. and McLemore, S. D. (1967). *Sociological Measurement: An Inventory of Scales and Indices*; Chandler Publishing Co., San Francisco, California.

Bower, J. D., Ackerman, P. G. and Toro, G. (1974). *Clinical Laboratory Methods*; 8th Edition, C. V. Mosby, St. Louis.

Catell, R. B. and Warburton, F. (1967). *Objective Personality and Motivation Tests: A Theoretical Introduction and Practical Compendium*; University of Illinois Press, Urbana.

Ciminero, A. R., Calhoun, K. S. and Adams, H. E. (eds) (1977). *Handbook of Behavioural Assessment*; Wiley, New York.

Chun, Ki-Taek, Cobb, S. and French, J. R. (1975). *Measures for Psychological Assessment: A Guide to 3,000 Original Sources and Their Applications*; Institute for Social Research, Ann Arbor, Michigan.

Comrey, A. L., Backer, T. E. and Glaser, E. M. (1973). *A Sourcebook for Mental Health Measures*; Human Interaction Research Institute, Los Angeles, California.

Cromwell, L., Weibell, F. J. and Pfeiffer, E. A. (1980). *Biomedical Instrumentation and Measurements*; 2nd Edition, Prentice Hall, Englewood Cliffs, New Jersey.

Ferris, C. (1980). *A Guide to Medical Laboratory Instruments*; Little Brown and Co., Boston.

Geddes, L. A. and Baker, L. E. (1975). *Principles of Applied Biomedical Instrumentation*; Wiley, New York.

General Practice Research Unit (1969). *General Health Questionnaire*; The NFER – Nelson Publishing Co., Windsor, Berks.

Goldman, B. A. and Saunders, J. L. (1974). *Directory of Unpublished Experimental Measures*; Vol I, Behavioural Publications, New York.

Goldman, B. A. and Saunders, J. L. (1978). *Directory of Unpublished Experimental Measures*; Vol II, Behavioural Publications, New York.

Haussmann, R. K. D., Hegyvary, S. T. and Newman, J. F. (1976). *The Rush-Medicus-Monitoring Methodology: Monitoring Quality of Nursing Care, Part 2 – Assessment and Study of Correlates*; DHEW Publication HRA 76–7, US Government Printing Office, Washington DC.

Jacox, A. K., Prescott, P. A., Collar, K. and Goodwin, L. D. (1981). *The Nurse Practitioner Rating Form: A Primary Care Process Measure*; Nursing Resources, Wakefield, Mass.

Johnson, O. G. (1976). *Tests and Measurements in Child Development*; Handbook II, Volumes 1 and 2, Jossey Bass, San Francisco, California.

Johnson, O. G. and Commarito, J. W. (1971). *Tests and Measurements in Child Development*; Handbook I, Jossey Bass, San Francisco, California.

Lake, D. G., Miles, M. B. and Earle, R. B. (1973). *Measuring Behaviour*; Teachers' College Press, New York.

Lyerly, S. (1973). *Handbook of Psychiatric Rating Scales*; 2nd Edition, National Institutes of Mental Health, Rockville, Maryland.

Miller, D. C. (1977). *Handbook of Research Design and Social Measurement*; 3rd Edition, David McKay, New York.

Pfeiffer, W. J., Heslen, R. and Jones, J. E. (1976). *Instrumentation in Human Relations Training*; 2nd Edition, University Associates, La Jolla, California.

Phaneuf, M. C. (1976). *The Nursing Audit: Self-regulation of Nursing Practice*; Appleton-Century-Crofts, New York.

Price, J. L. (1972). *Handbook of Organisational Measurement*; D. C. Heath, Lexington, Mass.

Reeder, L. G., Ramacher, L. and Gorelnik, S. (1976). *Handbook of Scales and Indices of Health Behaviour*; Goodyear, Pacific Palisades, California.

Robinson, J. P., Athanasiou, R. and Head, K. B. (1969). *Measures of Occupational Attitudes and Occupational Characteristics*; Institute for Social Research, University of Michigan, Ann Arbor, Michigan.

Robinson, J. P. and Shaver, P. R. (1973). *Measures of Social Psychological Attitudes*; Institute for Social Research, University of Michigan, Ann Arbor, Michigan.

Shaw, M. E. and Wright, J. M. (1967). *Scales for the Measurement of Attitudes*; McGraw Hill, New York.

Strauss, M. A. and Brown, B. W. (1978). *Family Measurement Techniques – Abstracts of Published Instruments 1935–1974*; Revised Edition, University of Minnesota Press, Minneapolis.

Wandelt, A. and Ager, J. (1975). *Quality Patient Care Scale (Qualpacs)*; Appleton-Century-Crofts, New York.

Wandelt, A. and Stewart, D. S. (1975). *Slater Nursing Competencies Rating Scale*; Appleton-Century-Crofts, New York.

Ward, M. J. and Felter, M. E. (1979). *Instruments for Use in Nursing Education Research*; Western Interstate Commission for Higher Education, Boulder, Colorado.

Weiss, M. (1973). *Biomedical Instrumentation*; Chilton Book Co., Philadelphia.

9 USEFUL ADDRESSES AND SOURCES OF INFORMATION

Department of Health Library,
Alexander Fleming House,
London,
SE1 6BY

English National Board for Nursing, Midwifery and Health Visiting,
Victory House,
170 Tottenham Court Road,
London,
WIP 0HA

English National Board for Nursing, Midwifery and Health Visiting,
Learning Resources Unit,
Chantrey House,
789 Chesterfield Road,
Sheffield,
S8 0SF

King's Fund Centre Library,
126 Albert Street,
London,
NW1 7NF

Royal College of Nursing Library,
20 Cavendish Square,
London,
W1M 0AB
(The Royal College of Nursing Library also houses the Steinberg
Collection of United Kingdom and North American Nursing Theses
and Dissertations.)

United Kingdom Central Council for Nursing, Midwifery and Health
Visiting,
23 Portland Place,
London,
W1N 3AF

✦ BIBLIOGRAPHY

RECOMMENDED FURTHER READING

Abrahams, P. (1982). *Historical Sociology*; Open Books, Shepton Mallet.

Agar, M. (1980). *The Professional Stranger: an Informal Introduction to Ethnography*; Academic Press, New York.

Agar, M. H. (1986). *Speaking of Ethnography*; Sage, Beverly Hills, California.

Altman, D. G., Gore, S. M., Gardner, M. J. and Pocock, S. J. (1983). Statistical Guidelines for Contributors to Medical Journals; *British Medical Journal*, **286**, 1489–93.

Anastasi, A. (1988). *Psychological Testing*; 6th Edition, Macmillan, New York.

Ashworth, P. D., Giorgi, A. and de Koning, A. J. J. (eds) (1986). *Qualitative Research in Psychology: Proceedings of the International Association for Qualitative Research*; Duquesne University Press, Pittsburgh, Pennsylvania.

Atkinson, P. (1981). *The Clinical Experience*; Gower, Farnborough, Hampshire.

Babbie, E. (1983). *The Practice of Social Research*; 3rd Edition, Wadsworth, Belmont, California.

Ball, M. J. and Hannah, K. J. (1984). *Using Computers in Nursing*; Reston Publishing, Reston.

Ball, S. J. (1983). Case Study Research in Education—Some Notes and Problems; in M. Hammersley (ed) (1983). *The Ethnography of Schooling: Methodological Issues*; Nafferton Books, Driffield, Humberside.

Barhyte, D. and Bacon, L. D. (1985). Approaches to Cleaning Data Sets: A Technical Comment; *Nursing Research*, **34**, 62–4.

Bayliss, D. (1983). Statistics for Nurses; *Nursing Times*, **79**, 47–50.

Bell, C. and Newby, H. (eds) (1977). *Doing Sociological Research*; Allen and Unwin, London.

Bell, J. (1987). *Doing Your Research Project: A Guide for First-Time Researchers in Education and Social Science*; Open University, Milton Keynes.

Belson, W. A. (1981). *The Design and Understanding of Survey Questions*; Gower, Aldershot.

Berelson, B. (1971). *Content Analysis in Communication Research*; Free Press, New York.

Borzak, L. (ed) (1981). *Field Study: a Sourcebook for Experimental Learning*; Sage, Beverly Hills, California.

Brenner, M., Brown, J. and Canter, D. (1985). *The Research Interview: Uses and Approaches*; Academic Press, London.

Brinberg, D. and McGrath, J. E. (1985). *Validity and the Research Process*; Sage, Beverly Hills, California.

British Museum, *General Catalogue of Printed Books*; British Museum, London.

British Psychological Society (1978). *Statement on Ethical Principles for Research with Human Subjects*; BPS, Leicester.

British Standards Institute (1978). *Recommendations for Citing Publications by Bibliographic References*; London.

Brooking, J. (ed) (1986). *Psychiatric Nursing Research*; John Wiley and Sons, Chichester.

Bryman, A. (1984). The Debate About Quantitative and Qualitative Research: a question of method or epistemology?; *British Journal of Sociology*, 35, 65–92.

Bryman, A. (1988). *Quantity and Quality in Social Research*; Unwin Hyman, London.

Bryman, A. (ed) (1988). *Doing Research in Organisations*; Routledge, London.

Burcham, W. E. and Rutherford, R. J. D. (eds) (1987). *Writing Applications for Research Grants*; 2nd Edition, Educational Development Advisory Committee, Occasional Publications No. 3, University of Birmingham.

Burgess, R. G. (1984). *In the Field: An Introduction to Field Research*; George Allen & Unwin, London.

Cahoon, M. C. (ed) (1987). *Research Methodology*; Recent Advances in Nursing Series, 17, Churchill Livingstone, Edinburgh.

Calnan, J. (1976). *One Way to Do Research: The A–Z for those who Must*; Heinemann, London.

Calnan, J. (1984). *Coping With Research: the Complete Guide for Beginners*; Heinemann, London.

Canter, D. (ed) (1985). *Facet Theory: Approaches to Social Research*; Springer-Verlag, New York.

Canter, D., Brown, J., and Groat, L. (1985). A Multiple Sorting Procedure for Studying Conceptual Systems; in Brenner, M., Brown, J., and Canter, D. (1985). *The Research Interview: Uses and*

Approaches; Academic Press, London, p. 79–114.

Chenitz, W. C. and Swanson, J. M. (1986). *From Practice to Grounded Theory: Qualitative Research in Nursing*; Addison Wesley, Menlo Park, New York.

Clark, J. M. and Hockey, L. (1979). *Research for Nursing: A Guide for the Enquiring Nurse*; HM and M, Aylesbury.

Converse, J. M. and Presser, S. (1986). *Survey Questions: Handcrafting the Standardised Questionnaire*; Sage, Beverly Hills.

Cook, T. D. and Reichardt, C. S. (1979). *Qualitative Methods in Evaluation Research*; Sage, Beverly Hills, California.

Cormack, D. F. S. (ed) (1984). *The Research Process in Nursing*; Blackwell, Oxford.

Cronbach, L. J. (1984). *Essentials of Psychological Testing*; 4th Edition, Harper and Row, New York.

Darling, V. H. and Rogers, J. (1986). *Research For Practising Nurses*; Macmillan, Basingstoke.

Davis, A. J. (1985). Ethical Issues in Nursing Research; *Western Journal of Nursing Research*, 7, 125–6.

Davis, B. D. (1983). *Research into Nurse Education*; Croom Helm, London.

De Vaus, D. A. (1986). *Surveys in Social Research*; George Allen & Unwin, London.

De Vellis, B. N., Adams, J. L. and De Vellis, R. F. (1984). Effects of Information on Patient Stereotyping; *Research in Nursing and Health*, 7, 237–44.

Deising, P. (1971). *Patterns of Discovery in the Social Sciences*; Aldine, New York.

Dempsey, P. A. and Dempsey, A. D. (1986). *The Research Process in Nursing*; Jones and Bartlett, Boston.

Dennis, K. E. (1986). Q Methodology: Relevance and Application to Nursing Research; *Advances in Nursing Science*, 8, 6–17.

Denzin, N. K. (1973). *The Research Act: A Theoretical Introduction to Sociological Methods*; Aldine, New York.

Denzin, N. K. (1978). *Sociological Methods: A Sourcebook*; 2nd Edition, McGraw Hill, New York.

Dilman, D. (1978). *Mail and Telephone Surveys: The Total Design Method*; Wiley, New York.

Dissertation Abstracts International, Ann Arbor, Michigan.

Dixon, B. R., Bouma, G. D. and Atkinson, G. B. J. (1987). *A Handbook of Social Science Research: A Comprehensive and Practical Guide for Students*; Oxford University Press, Oxford.

Dolst, D. F. and Hungler, B. P. (1985). *Essentials of Nursing Research*; Lippincott, Philadelphia.

Douglas, J. (1976). *Investigative Social Research*; Sage, Beverly Hills, California.

Dowrick, P. and Briggs, S. J. (eds) (1983). *Using Video: Psychological and Social Applications*; John Wiley and Sons, New York.

Duffy, M. E. (1985). Designing Nursing Research: The Qualitative-Quantitative Debate; *Journal of Advanced Nursing*, **10**, 225–31.

Feyerbend, P. (1978). *Against Method*; Varo, London.

Field, P. A. and Morse, J. M. (1985). *Nursing Research: The Application of Qualitative Approaches*; Croom Helm, London.

Fielding, N. G. and Fielding, J. L. (1985). *Linking Data*; Sage, Beverly Hills, California.

Filstead, W. J. (1970). *Qualitative Methodology: Firsthand Involvement With the Social World*; Rand McNally, Chicago.

Fink, A. and Kosekoff, J. (1985). *How to Conduct Surveys: A Step-by-Step Guide*; Sage, Beverly Hills, California.

Flanagan, J. C. (1954). The Critical Incident Technique; *Psychological Bulletin*, 51, **4**, 327–58.

Fox, D. J. (1982). *Fundamentals of Research in Nursing*; 4th Edition, Appleton-Century-Crofts, Norwalk, New Jersey.

Gardner, G. (1978). *Social Surveys for Social Planners*; Open University Press, Milton Keynes.

George, T. B. (1982). Development of the Self-Concept of Nurse in Nursing Students; *Research in Nursing and Health*, 5, 191–97.

Glaser, B. G. (1978). *Theoretical Sensitivity: Advances in the Methodology of Grounded Theory*; Sociology Press, Mill Valley, California.

Glaser, B. G. and Strauss, A. L. (1967). *The Discovery of Grounded Theory*; Aldine, New York.

Godsmith, J. W. (1981). Methodological Considerations in Using Videotape to Establish Rater Reliability; *Nursing Research*, 30, 124–7.

Goodwin, L. and Goodwin, W. (1984). Qualitative vs Quantitative Research or Qualitative and Quantitative Research?; *Nursing Research*, 33, 378–80.

Groat, L. (1982). Meaning in Post-Modern Architecture: An Examination Using The Multiple Sorting Task; *Journal of Environmental Psychology*, 2, 3–22.

Hakim, C. (1987). *Research Design: Strategies and Choices in the Design of Social Research*; George Allen & Unwin, London.

Hammersley, M. and Atkinson, P. (1983). *Ethnography: Principles in Practice*; Tavistock, London.

Hannah, K., Guillemin, F. and Conklin, D. N. (1986). *Nursing Uses of Computers and Information Science*; North Holland, Amsterdam.

Harris, R. B. and Hyman, R. B. (1984). Clean vs. Sterile Tracheotomy Care and Level of Pulmonary Infection; *Nursing Research*, 33, 80–5.

Hastings, E. H. and Hastings, P. K. (eds) (1980). *Index to International Public Opinion 1978–1979*; Greenwood Press, Westport, Connecticut.

Henshaw, A. and Schepp, K. (1984). Problems in Doing Nursing Research. How to Recognise Garbage When You See It!; *Western Journal of Nursing*, 6, 126–30.

Hockey, L. (1985). *Nursing Research: Mistakes and Misconceptions*; Churchill Livingstone, Edinburgh.

Hoinville, G., Jowell, R. and associates (1978). *Survey Research Practice*; Heinemann, London.

Howard, K. and Sharp, J. A. (1983). *The Management of a Student Research Project*; Gower, Aldershot.

Jacobson, S. F. (1983). Stresses and Coping Strategies of Neonatal Intensive Care Unit Nurses; *Research in Nursing and Health*, 6, 33–40.

Jacobson, S. F. (1984). A semantic differential for external comparison of conceptual nursing models; *Advances in Nursing Science*, 6, 58–70.

Kerlinger, F. N. (1986). *Foundations of Behavioural Research*; 3rd Edition, CBS Publishing, New York.

Kirk, J. and Miller, M. L. (1985). *Reliability and Validity in Qualitative Research*; Sage, Beverly Hills, California.

Knaak, P. (1984). Phenomenological Research; *Western Journal of Nursing Research*, 6, 107–14.

Knafl, K. A. and Howard, M. J. (1984). Interpreting and Reporting Qualitative Research; *Research in Nursing and Health*, 7, 17–24.

Kogan, M. and Henkely, M. (1983). *Government and Research: The Rothschild Experiment in a Government Department*; Heinemann, London.

Kovacs, A. R. (1985). *The Research Process: Essentials of Skill Development;* F. A. Davis, Philadelphia.

Krampitz, S. D. and Pavlovich, N. (1981). *Readings for Nursing Research*; C. V. Mosby, St Louis.

Krippendorff, K. (1980). *Content Analysis: an Introduction to Its Methodology*; Sage, Beverly Hills, California.

Leininger, M. M. (ed) (1985). *Qualitative Research Methods in Nursing*; Grune & Stratton, New York.

Macleod Clark, J. and Hockey, L. (1979). *Research for Nursing: A Guide for the Enquiring Nurse*; H. M. and M., London.

Manis, J. G. and Meltzer, B. N. (1978). *Symbolic Interaction*; Allyn and Bacon, Boston.

Marsh, C. (1982). *The Survey Method*; George Allen & Unwin, London.

Marshall, L. A. and Rowland, F. (1983). *A Guide to Learning Independently*; Open University Press, Milton Keynes.

Martin, P. Y. and Turner, B. A. (1986). Grounded Theory and Organisational Research; *Journal of Applied Behavioural Science*, 22, 141–58.

Mishel, M. H. (1981). The measurement of uncertainty in illness; *Nursing Research*, 30, 258–63.

Moyser, G. and Wagstaffe, M. (eds) (1987). *Research Methods for Elite Studies*; Allen and Unwin, London.

Notter, L. E. (1979). *Essentials of Nursing Research*; 2nd Edition, Tavistock, London.

Oiler, C. (1982). The Phenomenological Approach in Nursing Research; *Nursing Research*, 31, 178–81.

Oppenheim, A. N. (1966). *Questionnaire Design and Attitude Measurement*; Heinemann, London.

Osgood, C. E., Suci, G. J. and Tannenbaum, P. H. (1957). *The Measurement of Meaning*; University of Illinois Press, Urbana.

Paradoo, K. and Reid, N. (1988). Research Skills Number 1, Getting Started: The language of research; *Nursing Times*, 84, 39, 67–70.

Polit, D. F. and Hungler, B. P. (1987). *Nursing Research: Principles and Methods*; 3rd Edition, J. B. Lipincott, Philadelphia.

Popper, K. R. (1959). *The Logic of Scientific Method*; Hutchinson, London.

Research in British Universities, Polytechnics and Colleges; British Library, London.

Roberts, H. (ed) (1981). *Doing Feminist Research*; Routledge and Kegan Paul, London.

Rowntree, D. (1981). *Statistics Without Tears*; Penguin, London.

SSPS Inc (1983). *SPSS User's Guide*; McGraw Hill, New York.

Science Citation Index; Institute for Scientific Information, Philadelphia. Published three times a year.

Shipman, M. (1981). *The Limitations of Social Research*; 2nd Edition, Longmans, London.

Shye, S. (ed) (1978). *Theory Construction and Data Analysis in the Behavioural Sciences*; Jossey Bass, San Francisco.

Skevington, S. (ed) (1984). *Understanding Nurses: The Social Psychology of Nursing*; Wiley, Chichester.

Silverman, D. (1985). *Qualitative Methodology in Sociology*; Gower, Aldershot.

Social Science Citation Index; Institute for Scientific Information, Philadelphia. Published three times a year.

Sommer, R. and Sommer, B. B. (1980). *A Practical Guide to Behavioural Research: Tools and Techniques*; Oxford University Press, New York.

Spilker, B. (1984). *A Guide to Clinical Studies and Developing Protocols*; Raven Press, New York.

Spindler, G. (ed) (1982). *Doing the Ethnography of Schooling: Educational Anthropology in Action*; Holt, Rinehart and Winston, New York.

Spradley, J. A. (1980). *Participant Observation*; Holt, Rinehart and Winston, New York.

Strauss, A. L. (1987). *Qualitative Data Analysis for Social Scientists*; Cambridge University Press, Cambridge.

Sudman, S. and Bradburn, N. M. (1982). *Asking Questions: A Practical Guide to Questionnaire Design*; Jossey Bass, San Francisco.

Sudman, S. and Lannom, L. B. (1980). *Health Care Surveys Using Diaries*; NCHSR Research Report 80–84, National Center for Health Services Research, Hyattsville, Maryland.

Swanson, J. M. and Chenitz, W. C. (1982). Why Qualitative Research in Nursing?; *Nursing Outlook*, 30, 241–5.

Sweeney, M. A. (1985). *The Nurse's Guide to Computers*; Macmillan, New York.

Taylor, S. J. and Bogdan, R. (1984). *Introduction to Qualitative Research Methods: The Search for Meanings*; 2nd Edition, Wiley, New York.

Tornquist, E. M. (1986). *From Proposal to Publication: An Informal Guide to Writing About Nursing Research*; Addison Wesley, Menlo Park, New York.

Treece, E. W. and Treece, J. W. Jr. (1986). *Elements of Research in Nursing*; 4th Edition, Mosby, St. Louis.

Turabian, K. L. (1973). *A Manual for Writers of Term Papers, Theses and Dissertations*; 4th Edition, University of Chicago Press, Chicago.

Turner, B. A. (1981). Some Practical Aspects of Qualitative Data Analysis. One Way of Organising Some of the Cognitive Processes Associated with the Generation of Grounded Theory; *Quality and Quantity*, 15, 225–47.

United Nations Statistical Year Book; United Nations, New York. Published annually.

United States Library of Congress: The National Union Catalogue; Boston, Mass.

Van Maanen, J. (1983). *Qualitative Methodology*; Sage, Beverly Hills, California.

Van Zuuren, F. J., Wertz, F. J., and Mook, B. (1987). *Advances in Qualitative Psychology: Themes and Variations*; Swets & Zeitlinger B.V., Lisse.

Walsh, R. (ed) (1985). *A Bibliography of Nursing Literature*; Vol. 3, Library Association Publishing, London.

Waltz, C. F. and Bausell, R. B. (1981). *Nursing Research: Design, Statistics and Computer Analysis*; F. A. Davis, Philadelphia.

Waltz, C. F., Strickland, O. L. and Lenz, E. R. (1984). *Measurement in Nursing Research*; F. A. Davis Company, Philadelphia.

Watson, J. (1985). *Nursing: Human Science and Human Care: A Theory of Nursing*; Appleton-Century-Crofts, Norwalk, Connecticut.

Wattley, L. A. and Muller, D. (1984). *Investigating Psychology: A Practical Approach for Nursing*; Harper and Row, London.

Wax, R. (1971). *Doing Fieldwork: Warnings and Advice*; University of Chicago Press, Chicago.

Wenger, G. C. (ed) (1987). *The Research Relationship*; Allen & Unwin, London.

White, J. H. (1984). The Relationship of Clinical Practice and Research; *Journal of Advanced Nursing*, 9, 181–7.

Whyte, W. F. (1955). *Street Corner Society*; 2nd Edition, University of Chicago Press, Chicago.

Wilson, H. S. (1985). *Research in Nursing*; Addison Wesley, Menlo Park, New York.

Winstead-Fry, P. (ed) (1986). *Case Studies in Nursing Theory*; National League for Nursing, New York.

Woods, N. F. (1988). *Nursing Research, A Learning Resource*; Mosby, St Louis.

Yin, R. (1984). *Case Study Research: Design and Methods*; Applied Social Research Series No 5, Sage, Beverly Hills, California.

Zelditch, M. Jr. (1969). Some Methodological Problems of Field Studies; in B. J. McCall, and J. L. Simmons (eds) (1969). *Issues in Participant Observation: A Text and Reader*; Addison Wesley, Menlo Park, California.

◆AUTHOR INDEX

◆ <u>SUBJECT INDEX</u>

histograms, 59
historical research, 35, 56
hypothesis, 30, 35, 44, 45

identifying methods, 35, 36
indexes, 90
individual beliefs, 32
instruments, 53, 91–2
Inter-Library Loan system, 6, 21
interpreting data, 10
interval scales, 59
interview, 36
inventories, 53

journals, 56
  nursing, 8, 89

King's Fund Centre Library, 93

laws, 44
literature
  locating, 9
  resources, 85
  review, writing a, 26
  searching, 20–7

management of time, 65–6
mean, 59, 60
median, 59, 60
methodology, research, 28–33
mode, 59
multiple sorting, 36, 48, 52

negotiating access, 9
non-parametric tests, 59
non-participant observation, 47
normal distribution, 59
null hypothesis, 45
nurse educators, 2
nursing research
  examples of, 6–11
  topics, 6
nursing journals, 8

objectivity in research, 31
observation, 36, 40, 46, 47
open questions, 43
opportunistic sampling, 41
outlining, 66
overview of the research process, 4–11

parametric tests, 59
participant observation, 47
personal construct theory, 49
philosophical research, 35
physiological measures, 36
pie-charts, 59
pilot studies, 39
planning
  research project, 9, 12, 66
  report, 69–70
predictions, 30
preparing a research proposal, 9
presenting findings, 10
problems, clarifying, 12
programs, computer, 82–4
projective techniques, 36
proposal, writing a research, 9, 15
Psychological Abstracts, 23
publication, writing for, 72
purposive sampling, 41

Q sort, 36
qualitative analysis, 58–62, 63–4
qualitative methods, 3
qualitative research, 28, 29, 58
quantitative methods, 3
quantitative research, 28, 29, 58
questionnaires, 36, 40, 43, 44, 51
questions, 43
quota sampling, 41
quoting references, 79–81

rating scales, 54
ratio scales, 59
RCN Library, 93
recommendations, 10
records, using existing, 36, 48, 51
reference system, card, 24
referencing, 79–81
reliability, 41
repertory grid technique, 36, 48, 49
report writing, 10
research
  definitions of, 4–11
  descriptive, 30
  design, 34–9
  experimental, 30
  historical, 35, 56
  philosophical, 35
research process, overview, 4–11
research proposal, 9, 15